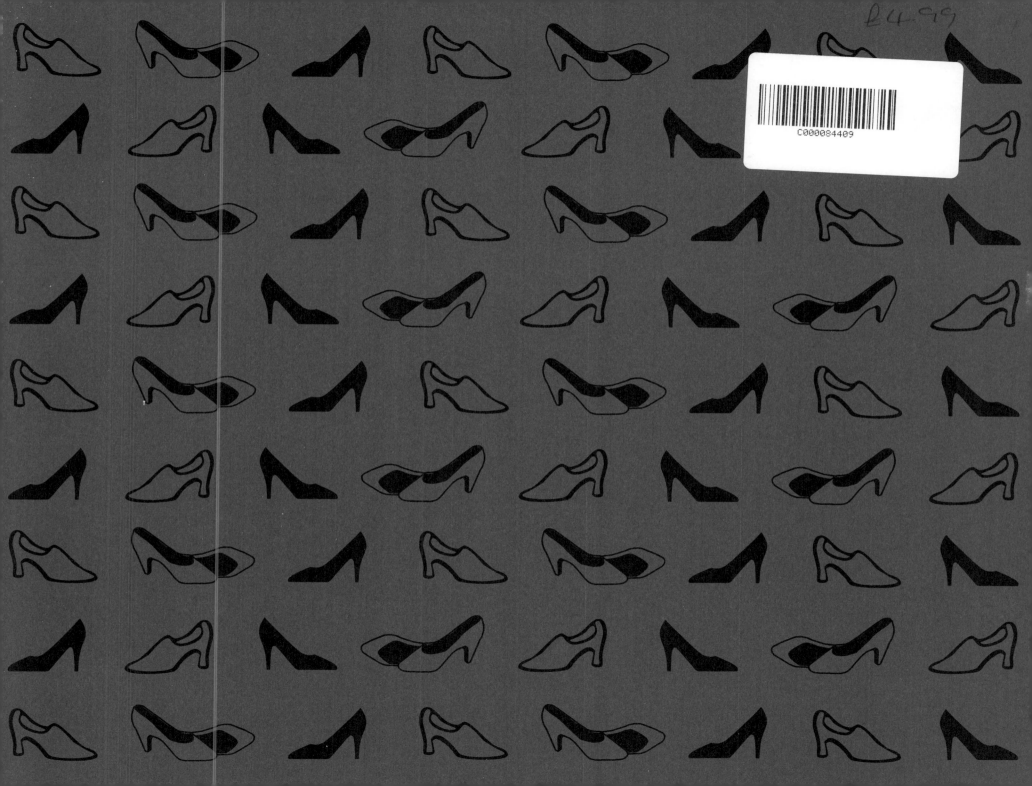

£4.99

C000084409

Hot Shoes

100 YEARS

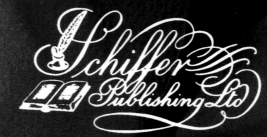

Maureen Reilly

Photography by John Klycinski

4880 Lower Valley Road, Atglen, PA 19310

Published by Schiffer Publishing, Ltd.
4880 Lower Valley Road
Atglen, PA 19310
Phone: (610) 593-1777; Fax: (610) 593-2002
E-mail: Schifferbk@aol.com
Please write for a free catalog.
This book may be purchased from the publisher.
Please include $3.95 for shipping.

In Europe Schiffer books are distributed by
Bushwood Books
6 Marksbury Avenue
Kew Gardens
Surrey TW9 4JF England
Phone: 44 (0) 181 392-8585; Fax: 44 (0) 181 392-9876
E-mail: Bushwd@aol.com

Please try your bookstore first.

We are interested in hearing from authors
with book ideas on related subjects.

Copyright © 1998 by Maureen Reilly
Library of Congress Catalog Card Number: 98-84561

All rights reserved. No part of this work may be reproduced or used in
any form or by any means—graphic, electronic, or mechanical, including
photocopying or information storage and retrieval systems—without
written permission from the copyright holder.

Designed by Blair Loughrey
Type set in Korinna BT

ISBN: 0-7643-0435-6
Printed in China

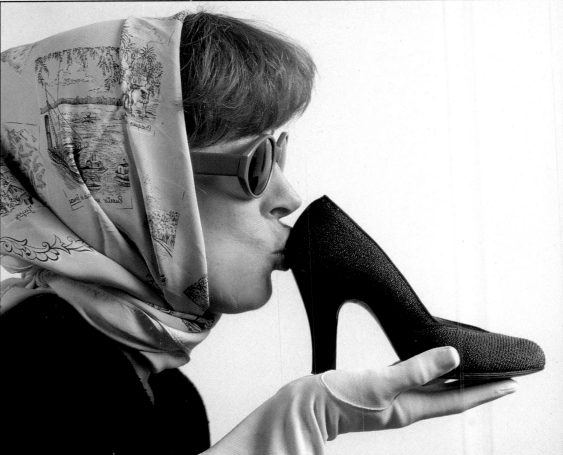

A perfect pair of pumps deserve a kiss! These, a diminutive size 4,
were fashioned from lacquered raffia by Palter De Liso, circa 1950.

TABLE OF CONTENTS

FIRST STEPS

This is a book for vintage shoe collectors, and all those who love fashion. More rational people may wonder why this particular subject has such allure. After all, shoes are shaped by the sweat of hard usage. They are pounded on pavement, spattered with mud, and soaked by rain. This abuse tells its own story, quite apart from the world of fashion.

When a china button is chipped, we wonder if the lady was impatient with her buttonhook. When a rhinestone buckle is loose, we can imagine a shoe kicked hastily aside during romantic dalliance. It is the essential earthiness of shoes that makes of them a touchstone to past lives and times.

What a powerful talisman is the shoe! Thankfully, many women pause before discarding a favorite pair, and take care to preserve it for the sake of memory. Often the prettiest shoes are barely worn and they emerge from closets still in their original boxes. When a wife swathes her bridal slippers in tissue, or a mother tucks away baby's first shoes in a lace-lined drawer, she seeks to connect the next generation to a past that is rich in personal history.

Of course, sometimes a shoe is just a shoe. Which is enough.

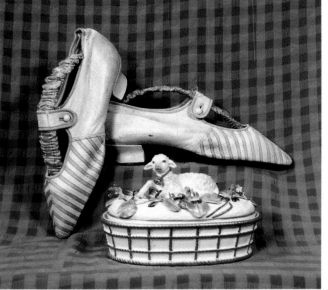

Slim grosgrain ribbons in a whisper-soft shade of celadon are stitched by hand in diagonal rows on dainty single-bar slippers. This detail, and the lamb-soft leather used to shape the uppers on straight soles, indicates that they were custom-made circa 1850. *Collection of Carol Sidlow.* Value: Special.

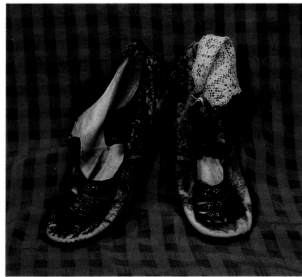

A pair of much-worn straights, circa 1840, in shattered kid, with low heels and marcasite trim. Shoemakers did not begin making soles shaped for left and right feet until the 1870s. *Courtesy of Lottie Ballou.* Value: Special.

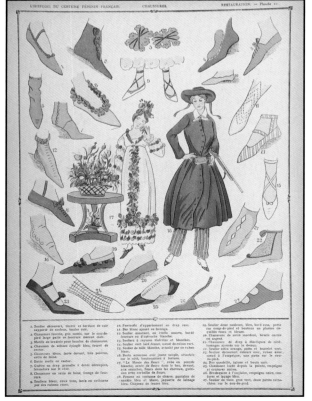

A bevy of straight-soled slippers from the Directoire period, following the French revolution. They were worn with diaphanous empire-waisted gowns. Some were so fragile as to require a daily coat of varnish! As shown in the hand-watercolored manuscript *L'Histoire du Costume Feminin Francais* by P. L. de Giafferi, published in France during the 1920s.

Shoes Last

STRAIGHTS

According to historians, the earliest shoes were cut to fit a left and right foot, which makes sense considering that these shoes were all custom-made. In the mid-1500s, cobblers began making soles in the same shape for either foot. These were called "straights." They didn't begin making lefts and rights again until the mid-1800s. This 300-year hiatus came to an end due to vanity or, more precisely, to the invention of high heels.

High heels are a modified version of the chopines worn by Venetian courtesans in the early 1500s. Chopines raised the sole of the shoe all over, something like the rafts that would be shown by Schiaparelli in the 1930s. Chopines were worn not just by ladies of the oldest profession, but also by the nobility, helping them to soar eighteen inches or more in height, so that servants had to assist with walking.

Somewhere along the line it was discovered that lowering the sole in front made it possible to walk without sacrificing height. The high heel was born by the late 1500s, and soon all of Europe was swept up in the newest style craze. But cobblers could not produce the enormous quantities of hand-turned wooden lasts required to arch the sole for a heel and then shape each last for a right and left foot. The choice between comfort and fashion was obvious, and society opted for the latter: heels on shoes that were not shaped, but straight.

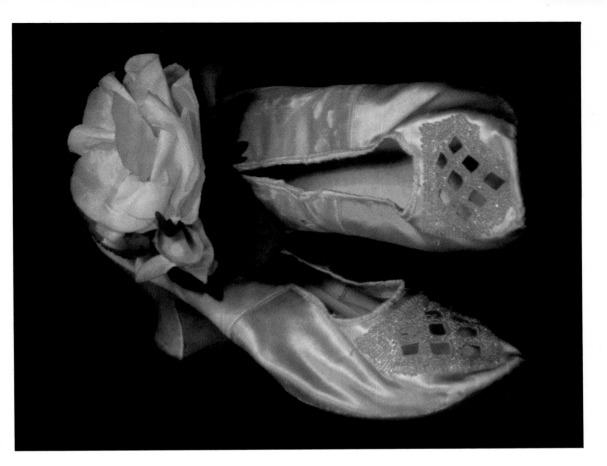

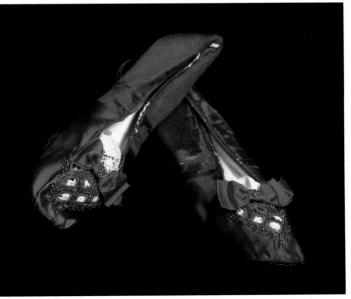

Above & Left: These lovely shoes seem to glow with an inner fire, like fine rubies and pearls. They are nearly straight of sole, with low-waisted Louis heels, circa 1870. Both feature diamond-shaped cut-work on the vamp, outlined in beads. As happens so often with shoes of this caliber, the owners can't bear to part with them, even though they are in the business of selling vintage clothing at their Los Angeles shop, Time After Time. *Collection of Jacquelyn and Mariusz Olbrychowski.* Value: Special.

5

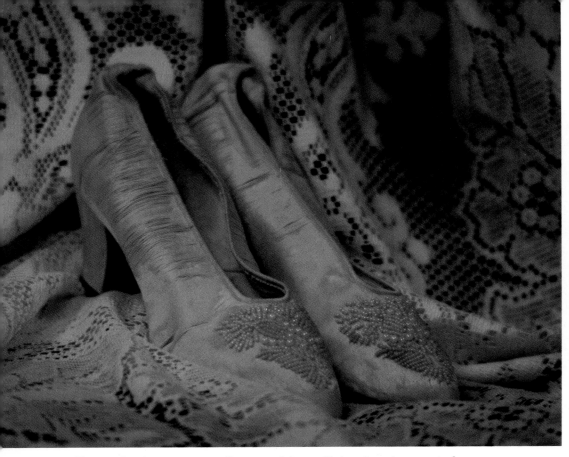

Shattered satin pumps are well-worn and thus unlikely to have been part of a bridal costume. These date to the Edwardian era, although they have the low heels and plain lines of pumps from the mid-1800s. However, they have a slight left and right distinction in the soles and pointed toes, which date them later. *Courtesy of The Blue Parrot.* Value: $95-115.

Ironically, straights were still made in the years following the French revolution. It was the Regency in England, the Directoire period in France. It was a period of simplicity in dress based on the ancient Greek ideal, when shoes were plain and flat. Perhaps it was just a matter of habit by this time to wear straights, because they continued in use, even when there was no need for an arched heel last per foot. In any event, by the 1870s the cobbler's craft caught up with his art. About the time of the American Civil War, lasts were being produced in factories and shoemakers were finally, once again, cutting a different sole for the left and right foot.

In the United States, we know that the first set of left and right lasts was made by William Young of Philadelphia, and sold to the Daniel Silsbee manufacturing company in 1822.

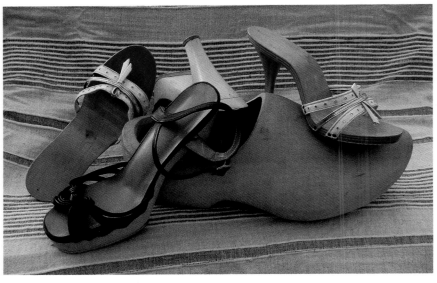

Wooden shoes have been the sturdy footwear of hard-working Europeans since the Middle Ages. They are still worn by farmers and fishermen throughout the Netherlands, Portugal, Spain, France, and Italy. Faced with the leather shortages of World War II, wooden *sabots* gained a new popularity in England as well. Perhaps inspired by those days of "make do and mend," designers continued to use wood for fashionable footwear. The cocktail mules were Made in Italy in the early '60s; the revival platforms are from the late '60s. *Courtesy of Lindy's Shoppe.* Value: $15-35.

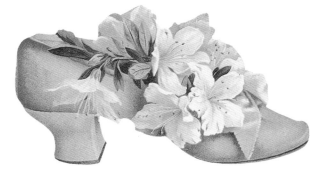

A sea-foam-blue silk court shoe of the seventeenth century, frothing with baroque whimsy. Note the low-waisted Louis heel, so named after the stylish Louis XV. It was about one-hundred years earlier that heels were first applied to shoes, for both sexes.

A CUSTOM FIT

Just how important was a custom fit for footwear that was sold in the middle decades of this century? If magazine ads are to be believed, it was critical. In June 1936, Foot Saver Shoes announced "The Fourth Dimension" in form with its "Shortback Foot Savers." The company's oxford and T-strap styles sold for $9-12.50, well worth the price considering that so much scientific testing went into their design:

"For a long time we knew something was wrong with women's shoes. They gapped at the sides, they pinched the toes, they wore out stockings. So we measured thousands of women's feet—first by length and then by parts—the parts from the toe to the ball and the ball to the heel. That's where we made a discovery: The modern woman's foot, regardless of its size, is actually shorter, in back, than most people realize. No wonder women have had to fill their shoes with heel pads or other gadgets to make them fit. Now you can get, in Shortback Foot Savers, a shoe that really fits. We've made your regular size but we've made the back part slightly shorter—and you'll thrill when you see and feel what a difference it makes!"

Not to be outdone, in April 1936, Bellaire's motto was "foot slenderizing." It advertised a unique custom fit. "A delight to wear for concealed air cushions gently massage your foot as you walk, stimulating healthy circulation, the secret of youthful foot slenderness." We're not sure about the slenderizing bit, but we agree that cushions mean extra comfort!

Along similar lines, Red Cross introduced a line of "fit-tested" shoes in August 1945:

"You can't buy a new Gold Cross Shoe style until it's Fit-Tested for weeks on active, human feet. Before any Gold Cross style is introduced, handmade originals are worn . . . walked in . . . for weeks. Checked, daily, by our designers for even a hint of gapping, wrinkling, binding. Changed. Checked again. Until the kind of fit is assured that millions of women tell you they find only in . . . America's famous Fit-Tested footwear."

Here are a few other examples of the focus on fit, from a random survey of vintage *Vogue* and *Harper's Bazaar* magazines:

• In April 1936, the M. N. Arnold Shoe Co. promised "variety and beauty . . . (in) the finest, mellowest leathers." Their perforated leather oxfords were rather pricey at $10.50, but perhaps the comfort was worth it, as "something you can hardly believe before you try on a pair."

• In June 1941, it was "Wings over Mexico" for a trio of open-toe pumps. "Designed and made by Palter De Liso on his exclusive Capri and Stratford lasts that outline the print of your foot. And moulded to your individual fit and comfort by the magic touch of 'Lastex' yarn."

• In April 1939, Gray Brothers of Syracuse advertised the Grayflex Trampers label with reference to the New York World's Fair: "History will probably record 1939 as America's 'Walk Year'. This is the year to make the permanent acquaintance of Grayflex Trampers—shoes so soft and flexible that walking becomes a pleasure." Priced at $6.75 to $7.75 for oxfords, ghillies, and spectator pumps.

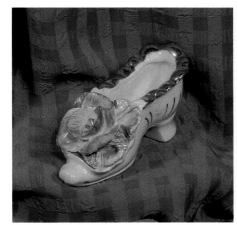

Ruffles are hand-painted in 14K gold on this fine china slipper. Court shoes like this were lavished with luxury detailing, for a shoemaker's "carriage trade" clientele. A real shoe of this caliber would have been formed on a custom last, followed by fittings. *Courtesy of Rich Man, Poor Man.* Value: $25.

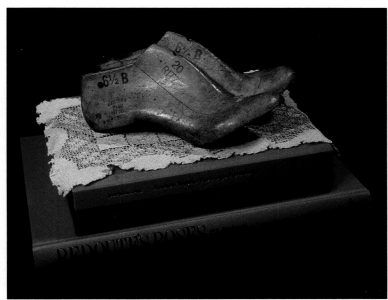

Throughout the first half of the century, in the days before mass production, shoe manufacturers sized their shoes on wooden molds such as this pair. The extended toe and flexed arch would have fit a size 6½ narrow on a 3-inch heel. The cobbler's craft excelled further for the carriage trade, such that each customer had a personalized last, to custom-fit each style to her own foot. You can find vintage shoe molds at antique stores and flea markets; expect to pay about $25-45 the pair. *Author's collection.*

- In May 1939, Red Cross boasted of "custom quality—custom fit—and at a surprising price." That price was $6.50 a pair for a wide range of perforated leather oxfords.

- In May 1949, the Irving Drew company advertised a bow-tied ghillie with three-inch heel as follows: "Custom-like craftsmanship . . . fine fit which only Drew shoemakers can impart . . . (and) exclusive Ankle-Fit features . . . Sculptured to Fit your Foot."

- In August 1949, Sandler of Boston featured moccasins in wedgie and Cuban-heeled styles. It assured that feet would be "resting in soft upper leather . . . wrapping in perfect fit . . . with hand-sewn vamps and backs." At $10.95 to $12.95.

- In September 1958 it was "the touch of Edith Henry . . . versatile flats and elegant little heeled shoes. In discovering the joy of (her) Lucky Strides and Whis-purrs, you'll find that size is really a pleasure because most styles come in sizes 2½ to 14, AAAAAAA to C, priced $7.95 to $12.95."

Imagine a manufacturer going to such lengths today! It used to be standard practice for shoes to come in many different widths at both heel and toe box. Also, made-to-order shoes were available in the ready-to-wear market through the 1950s. Now only the very wealthiest can afford such luxury.

Is it any wonder that shoe collectors often plan to wear their purchases, not so much for the vintage style as the custom fit? You can readily find any retro look, such as the stiletto revival of 1997, in vintage styles. Then there's the perennial oxford on sturdy Cuban heels to pair with pants. Or try mixing the lingerie look for evening with elegant hostess slippers from the 1940s. If you're squeamish about wearing previously worn shoes, look for new\old stock.

As you'll see throughout this book, vintage shoes were made from the finest leathers and fabrics. They often featured mesh inserts or elastic gores for coolness and ease of movement. They usually have inner cushions and supports, and the range of sizing is incredible. Try them on for a step in the right direction to comfort and style.

The excellence of Bally craftsmanship is evident in pale celadon linen pumps with python trim. *Courtesy of Lottie Ballou.* Value: $95-115.

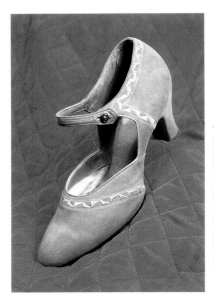

Two similar pairs by Bally in gray-green suede. Both this shoe, and the linen pair shown at left, have ziggurat stitching and mother-of-pearl buttons. *Author's collection.* Value: $75-95.

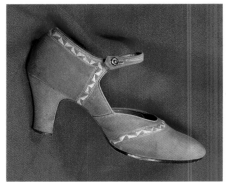

As recalled by the author's aunt, Mrs. Regina Glass, it was not unusual for the finer shoe salons in New York City to fit a last to their frequent customers. In the late '20s, she would order custom shoes each season in her choice of fabric, snakeskin, or suede.

Form is Function

It's hard to over-emphasize the impact of rubber as a new product on sport shoes and protective footwear. Without it, there would be no sneaker or rain boot or flip-flop. And without the comfort and flexibility of such shoes, it's hard to imagine the active lifestyle that has become a credo in all walks of life during the latter decades of this century.

> "Shoes are the only accessory you can't leave the house without."
> —Patrick Cox, 1997

THE SPORTING LIFE

In 1844 the American inventor Charles Goodrich patented a process for heat-treating rubber called "vulcanization." His method was used to make countless objects, from automobile tires, to life-preservers, to rubber-soled shoes and boots. It was not too long before canvas uppers and laces were added to the soles for the first sport shoe, dubbed the "croquet sandal." It proved so popular that it went into mass production—with the less elitist name of "sneaker"—and was marketed through the Sears Roebuck Catalog.

In 1917, the sneaker became an icon of American footwear when the U.S. Rubber Company produced them under the familiar Keds label (derived from "kids" and "ped"). The sneaker's basic style would not change for fifty years, until the invention of waffle-soled Nikes in 1972.

Rubber-soled shoes were also ideally suited for early bathing beauties, blending modesty with practicality at the beach or lake. (Women would continue to wear "bathing booties" well beyond the Victorian Era, into the 1920s and '30s.)

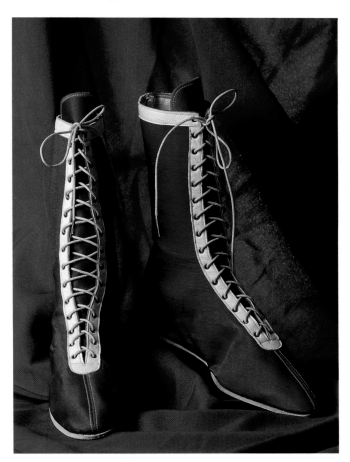

Left: High-laced wading shoes for a bathing beauty, circa 1920. They are fashioned from red satin and feature metal grommets. Clearly, these boots were meant for board-walking, not wading! With rubber soles stamped "Rautex," these are new\old stock from the N. B. Blackstone Co. in Los Angeles. They still bear an original price tag of $5.50. *Collection of Carol Sidlow.* Value: Special.

Below: Rubber wading shoes, circa 1930, sporting geometric trim in nautical blue. All forms of wearing apparel—and bathing costumes were no exception—incorporated streamlined design elements after the 1925 Paris Exposition *Internationale des Arts Decoratifs et Industriels Modernes. Collection of Sheryl Birkner.* Value: Special.

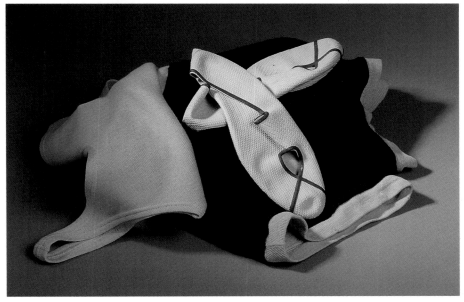

The footwear that American women have wished for

A wide variety of models in trim, stylish shoes—so reasonable you can afford a pair for practically every gown

THE shoes you have been waiting for. Fashionable footwear with all the newest lines, in the season's most popular fabric.

Models that are just right for every kind of wear—that are appropriate with practically every gown—and so inexpensive you can afford as many as you need.

Keds are made of finely woven canvas. The shapes are always right. The models are planned by expert designers who are well in touch with style tendencies for the coming season. There are shoes with half Louis heels, with military heels, with flat heels, and outing shoes with no heels at all. They fit snugly but are so flexible and light that they are most comfortable even in hot weather. The sport shoes are ideal for any kind of exercise—allowing the foot full freedom with just the right support.

This year the new models in Keds include shoes that are made just like leather shoes—welt construction soles, firmly boxed toes and the reinforcements that give the shoe body. It means a more formal, dignified shoe—a shoe that has the style of the most expensive leather shoes.

There are numerous pumps and oxfords and high shoes—suitable for street costume or the fluffiest of your frocks. There are very smart sport shoes—both high and low—trig enough for the dressiest tea at the Country Club. And then there are the heel-less tennis shoes, always so satisfactory for knock-about wear. Many women have found them wonderfully comfortable for house shoes. There are also shoes for men and boys for sport wear and for every day.

The children's Keds are made on the wide lasts that allow proper foot freedom. They are light and cool and give just the right protection for little feet.

Keds are made only by the United States Rubber Company. All the resources and experience of this company have been used in perfecting a line of stylish, practical shoes for all the family.

You will find Keds at every good shoe dealer's. Ask to see the various models. Notice how wonderfully light and comfortable they are—how trim your foot appears. Look at the models for the rest of the family. The name Keds is always a safeguard—on the sole of the shoe.

For men and women, $1.50 to $6.00
For children   1.15 to 4.50

United States Rubber Company

Keds

A STREET SHOE WITH THE NEWEST LINES
A full eight inches high for the new short skirts, these Keds have either a military heel or a half-Louis heel.

TO WEAR WITH THE FLUFFIEST FROCK
A trig little oxford with either a French or a military heel—graceful vamp—slender lines. These Keds have welt construction soles and firm inner supports.

FOR TWINKLING LITTLE FEET
Either in all white or in brown with smooth rubber soles to match. A full width model for growing feet. May be had with a welt construction sole. A similar Keds model has a corrugated sole and pump bow. In women's and misses' sizes also.

THE MOST POPULAR SPORT SHOES THE COUNTRY OVER
These shoes are being worn at all the fashionable resorts. Snugly fitting ankle, light and springy.

Trim and stylish canvas oxfords, meant for street wear in the summertime with the dressy touch of a stacked wooden heel, circa 1920. *Courtesy of Lottie Ballou.* Value: $45–65.

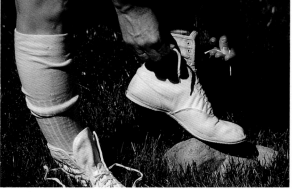

These "heel-less tennis shoes" bear the Keds logo, and are remarkably similar to the shoe in the lower right corner of the 1920 advertisement by that company, shown at far left. *Collection of Sheryl Birkner.* Value: Special.

Put on your high-button sneakers! Canvas shoes with rubber soles have been marketed by Keds since the late teens, soon after the process of bonding rubber to fabric was stabilized for commercial usage. As shown in this advertisement from the June 1920 issue of *The Designer and The Woman's Magazine,* some styles were "made just like leather shoes—welt construction soles, firmly boxed toes and the reinforcements that give the shoe body." Keds also offered sport shoes: "A trig little oxford with either a French or a military heel (and) the heel-less tennis shoes, always so satisfactory for knock-about wear."

The author's husband takes a well-deserved break. The original cleats were removed from his two-tone golf shoes, making them suitable for street wear. *Author's collection.* Value: Special.

STORMY WEATHER

Roman soldiers encased their sandals in leather for use in bad weather, based on a style of shoe worn by the subjugated Gauls. Centuries later, the Gaulish sandal gave its name to rubber galoshes! (Once again, rubber was used to assure sure footing in rain and sleet.) Another theory is that the name derives from "gal," the Roman word for wood and may be linked to the wood and iron pattens used to protect shoes.

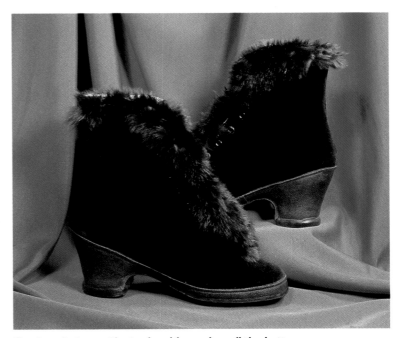

Suede galoshes, with sturdy rubber soles, all the better for splashing through puddles! By U.S. Gaytees, circa 1940. *Courtesy of Lottie Ballou.* Value: $25-45.

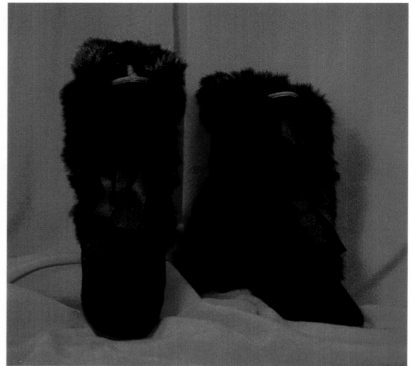

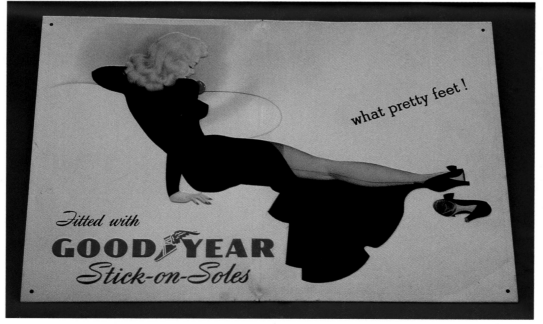

Above: Since early automobiles were open, protection from the cold was a necessity of motor travel. Ladies would don carriage boots like this cozy pair in fur-trimmed velvet, circa 1915 to 1925. They slipped on over regular shoes, and were not meant to be worn outside the vehicle. *Courtesy of the Blue Parrot.* Value: $195-225.

Left: In the 1930s and '40s, the U.S. Goodyear Co. made rubber soles that were widely sold in shoe repair shops, as advertised by this tin placard of a well-shod Vargas Girl.

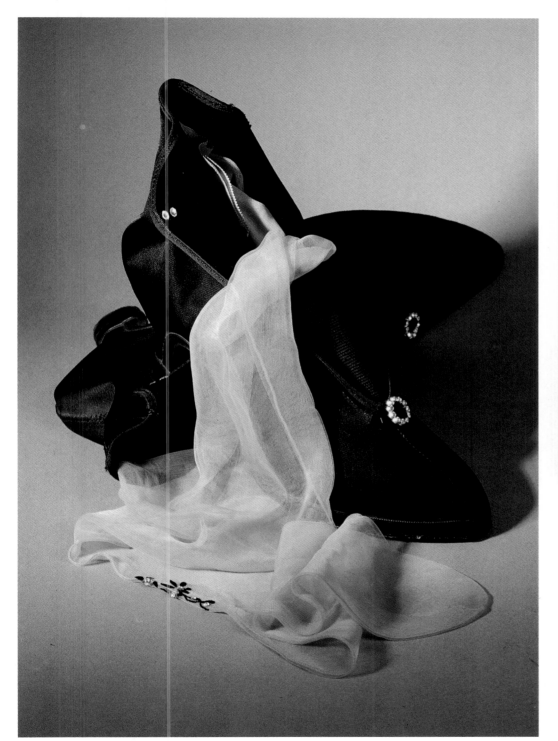

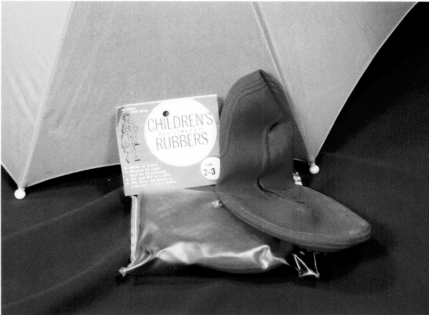

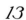

Above: Cheerful red rubbers for rainy schooldays, circa 1950, shown with the original clear display envelope for the Torch brand of Children's All Stretch Rubbers. *Courtesy of Lottie Ballou.* Value: $10-15.

13

Left: A well-shod woman of the 1930s and '40s would have had elegant rain boots for evening. Note the amusing ankle "pleat" that forms when the rhinestone buckles are clasped. The silk stockings with beaded clocks are from the '20s. *Boots courtesy of Pamela Joyce; stockings courtesy of Luxe.* Value: boots, $45-65; stockings, $35-55.

Chapter II

ELEMENTS OF DESIGN

Shoes are the one item of costume that must place function over form. Hems can rise or fall, hats can come or go, but shoes must conform to the shape of the foot, offer protection, and enable movement. This aspect of footwear has always created a compelling challenge for shoe designers. It has been said that "Shoes are the exclamation point at the end of a fashion statement."

The Form

We know the pump as a woman's shoe, but its origins may be traced to the masculine courtier or *court* shoe of the fifteenth century. Some fashion historians relate its basic design to the flat-heeled *pompe*, which was part of the uniform worn by footmen in the sixteenth century.

Of course, the earliest form of footwear was the sandal, as depicted in the hieroglyphs of ancient Egypt and the sculpture of classical Rome. When they were enclosed with leather, as required for warmth, the shoe was born.

In her autobiography, published in 1984, Diana Vreeland tells a wonderful story of how she brought the thong-toed leather sandal into fashion for day wear in this country. Mrs. Vreeland was a native-born American, but so traveled that she may as well have been a gypsy. Her sandal was discovered on a trip to the bordello district of ancient Pompeii, with lurid frescoes and certain ar-

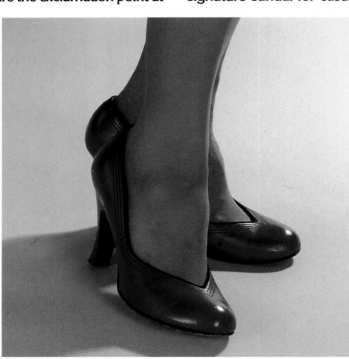

Given the pump's classic silhouette, color is a real focal point. Here, the spotlight is on red, accented with black cording on a sweetheart vamp. By Curvos, circa 1950. *Courtesy of Cheap Thrills*. Value: $25-35.

tifacts preserved for all time by the flow of lava. There, she claims to have noted a simple one-thong sandal with ankle-strap on the foot of an otherwise naked slave who had been thus frozen, in *flagrant delicto*. She commissioned the same design from a shoemaker and it became her signature sandal for casual wear. Mrs. Vreeland was a woman of great style and her vision would influence untold thousands of women during the years that she worked as fashion editor of *Harper's Bazaar* and then editor-in-chief of *Vogue* in the 1950s and '60s.

Let's explore these styles, and variations thereof, from the vantage point of vintage shoe collecting.

BASIC SHAPES

The shapes are pump, sandal, boot, slipper. But is there really any such thing as a basic shoe? If so, how come women can't seem to get enough of them in their closets?

Joan Crawford is reported to have owned 300 pairs; Jayne Mansfield, 200. These are measly numbers, compared to the 1,060 pairs totted up for Imelda Marcos. We can only speculate what Dolly Parton, Cher, and Madonna have spent on keeping their tootsies high and dry over the years.

One thing these ladies have in common, it would seem, is a shopping motto: "If the shoe fits, buy it!"

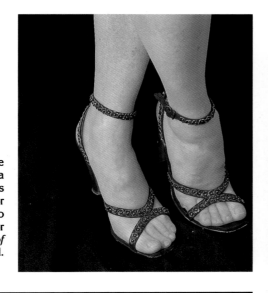

Bronze beading on brown suede sandals by Herbert Levine, circa 1960. The strippy straps of this pair cross the toe cleavage for sexy style, but sandals can also be the ultimate comfort shoe for daytime wear. *Collection of Pamela Joyce.* Value: Special.

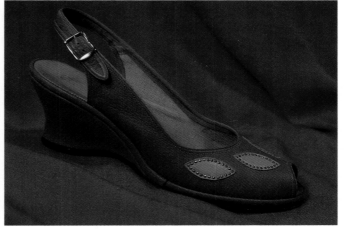

A sculpted wedgie from the late 1940s or early '50s, built for comfort as a casual slingback. In acorn brown with a studded leaf motif, ready for long walks in the fall woods. The label is Playarch, by Penaljo. *Author's collection.* Value: $15-25.

Daniel Green, a label well-known for slippers and "bridge shoes" in the '30s and '40s, later expanded to a line of dressy sandals. The pink bed slipper is "Powder Puff" priced at $7; the blue hostess mule is "Tiara" priced at $7.50; the two sandals with jeweled trim are only slightly higher in price, as advertised in 1955.

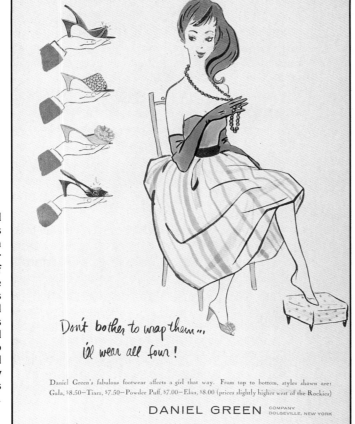

Don't bother to wrap them... i'll wear all four!

Daniel Green's fabulous footwear affects a girl that way. From top to bottom, styles shown are: Gala, $8.50—Tiara, $7.50—Powder Puff, $7.00—Elan, $8.00 (prices slightly higher west of the Rockies)

DANIEL GREEN COMPANY DOLGEVILLE, NEW YORK

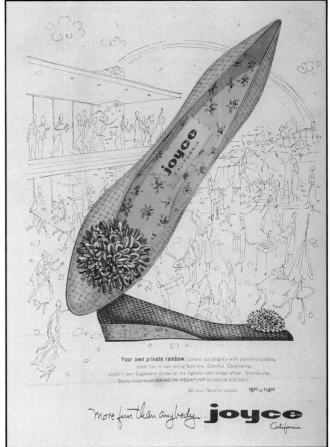

Your own private rainbow. Comes out brightly with polished cottons, other fun 'n sun loving fashions. Colorful. Captivating. Joyce's own Sugarcane Straw on the lightest cork wedge afloat. Spectacular. Styles illustrated: RAINBOW PEAKPUMP in natural and black.

All your favorite Joyces . . . $8⁹⁵ to $14⁹⁵

more fun than anybody ...joyce California

Joyce made slim wedgies for a summertime skimmer in 1958.

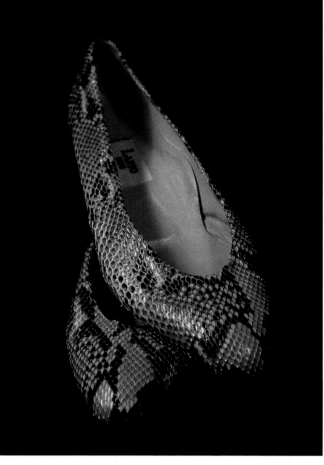

Right: If you must wear flats, make them chic flats, like the python pair shown to the left. These are by the semi-custom firm Lario, imported from Italy circa 1970. *Collection of Chris Cords.* Value: $75-95.

Below: The ballet flat is a pretty perennial. They first appeared as hostess wear when leather was in short supply during World War II and were soon adapted for everyday. This is the type of flat worn with Capri pants in the 1940s and '50s. In the '70s, it became the signature style of a new shoe company, Sam & Libby. *Author's collection.* Value: $10-15.

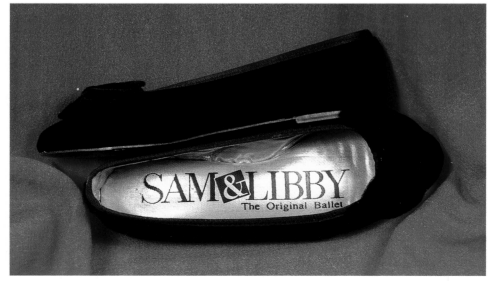

PUMPED

In the 1830s, Count Alfred Guillaume Gabriel d'Orsay refined the courtier's shoe for a woman's dainty foot. Quite the dandy, and a social maverick, he sculpted a new last with his own hands. It featured a V-shaped vamp and scalloped side. Then, as now, this pump was cut from kidskin on a low-slung, two-inch heel. Sexy like Bacall, elegant like Hepburn, that's the classic d'Orsay.

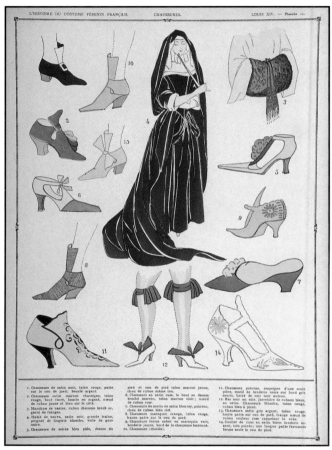

The pump is plain and classic in silhouette, derived from the courtier or "court" shoe in the days of King Louis XIV. The characteristic waisted heel and high vamp were charmingly illustrated and hand-watercolored in *L'histoire du Costume Feminin Francais* by P. L. Giafferri. We are not sure what the nun's habit has to do with footwear, however.

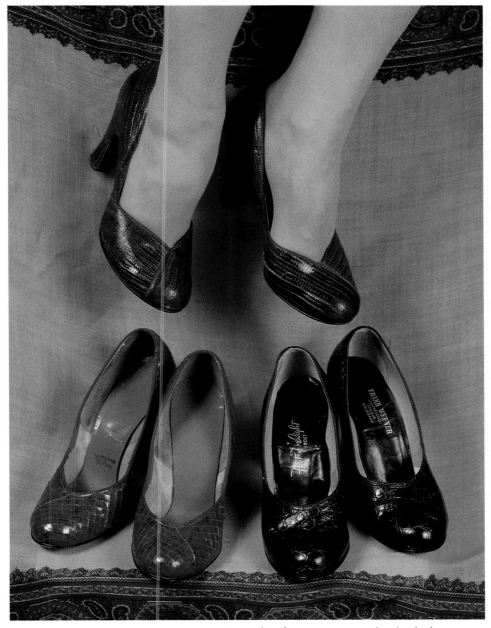

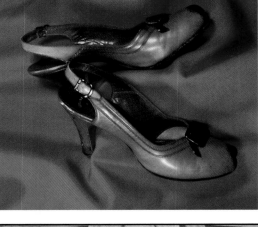

The pump becomes a slingback when its heel is cut out, and may be further modified for warm weather by a peep-toe as shown in this gray kid pair by De Liso Debs. These variations were developed in the late '20s. In prior years, a glimpse of heel or toe would have been too daring. *Courtesy of Lottie Ballou.* Value: $25-45.

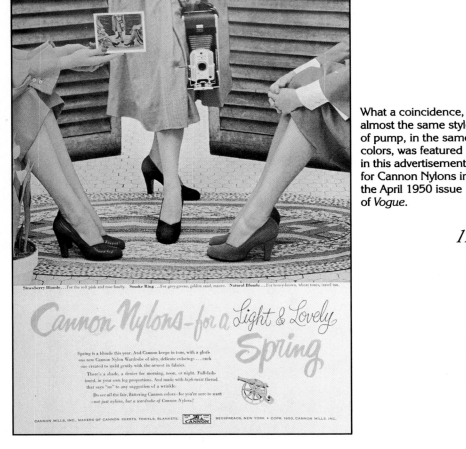

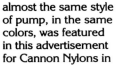

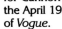

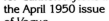

What a coincidence, almost the same style of pump, in the same colors, was featured in this advertisement for Cannon Nylons in the April 1950 issue of *Vogue*.

17

These well-cared for pumps were all obtained at the same estate sale, clearly the favorite style of some young woman in the late 1940s or early '50s. The red cobra is by DreamSteps, the green crocodile is by Foot Delight, and the brown snakeskin is from Filene's Basement in Boston. *Courtesy of Lottie Ballou.* Value: $65-95 each.

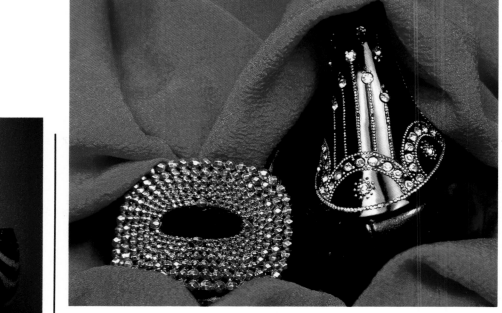

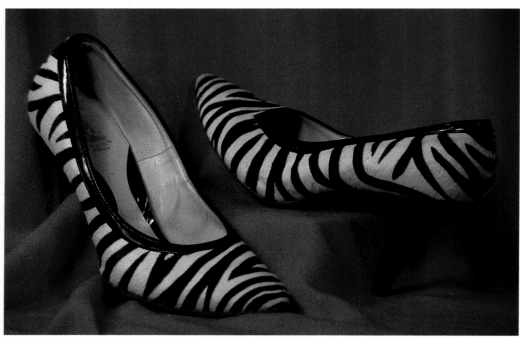

Walk on the wild side in faux zebra fur. These low-slung pumps were designed by Frank More for his Reno salon, circa 1960. *Courtesy of Luxe.* Value: $45-65.

Above: Stars falling in a night sky! It's a constellation of prong-set rhinestones and hand-painted beading on fabulous Bakelite heels. The cut-steel buckles on these dance pumps from the early '20s are a holdover from the Edwardian era. *Collection of Sylvia and Richard Unger.* Value: Special.

Right: Black suede swoops into a bow at the peep-toe of late 1940s slingbacks by Fenton for Saks Fifth Avenue. *Courtesy of Lottie Ballou.* Value: $35-55.

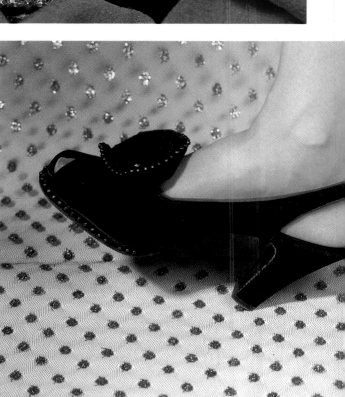

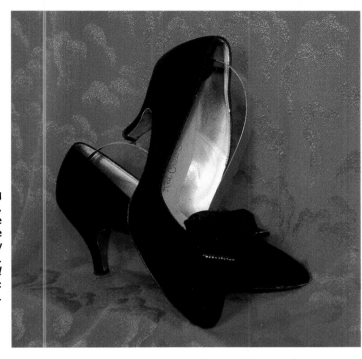

The evening pump, circa 1960, in black suede with rhinestone fans at the toe, by Red Cross. *Collection of Gail Pocock.* Value: Special.

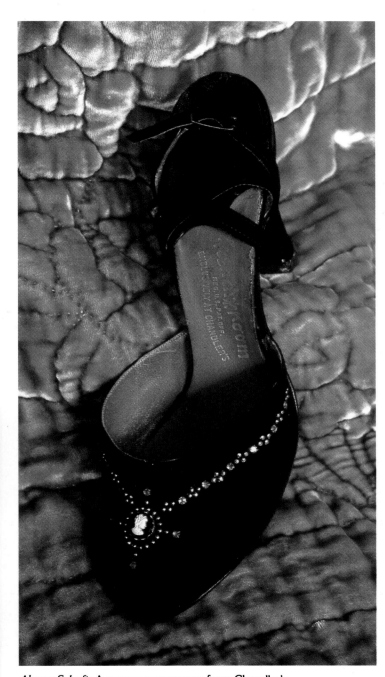
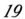

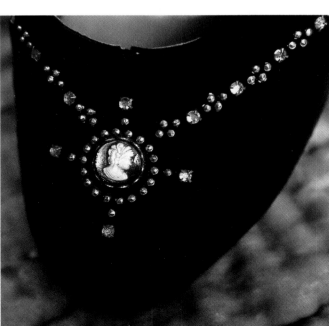

Above & Left: A cameo appearance from Chandler's French Room, circa 1960. Mock marcasite beading frames the delicate portrait, then radiates the vamp like a starburst. *Collection of Connie Beers.* Value: Special.

HEEL AND TOE

Foot Note on Heels: Louis XIV, the Sun King, was a sartorial sight to behold. As depicted in paintings, he favored towering ostrich-plume headdresses, short pantaloons puffed like a tutu, and garters emblazoned with golden sun rays. The problem was, his highness was a bit short. To compensate, he became a spokes model of sorts for heels. Louis XIV created a craze for men's heels as high as five inches, and the fun didn't stop there. His were decorated with miniature paintings of famous battles, or classical idylls. At the very least, they were covered in red leather. His courtiers soon copied red heels for their court shoes.

Carved Lucite heels and vinyl vamps were highly popular in the 1950s for making the rounds of post-war parties. Look for designer labels like Herbert Levine and Frank More; store labels like Chandlers, Reeves, and QualiCraft. As always, value depends on condition, but you can still find these shoes in the $25-55 range.

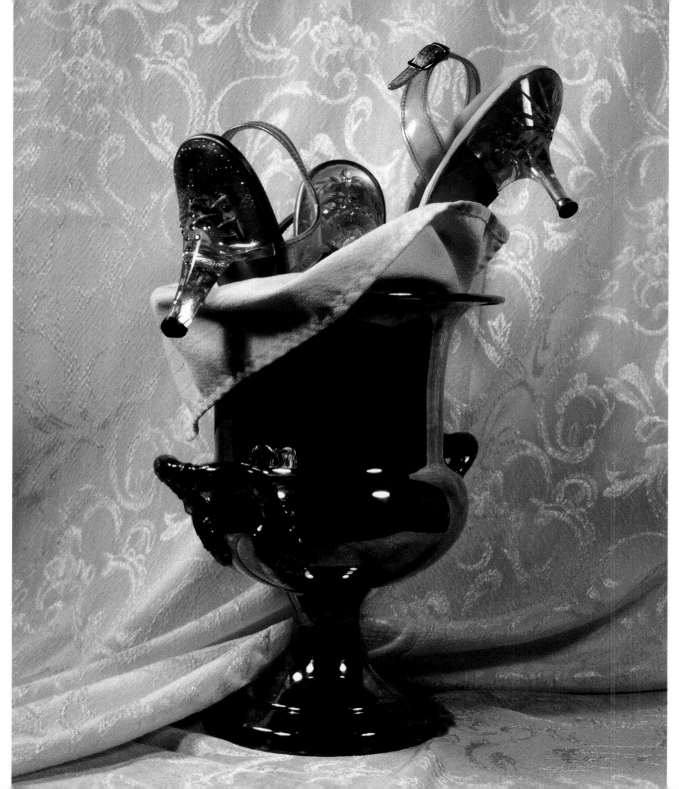

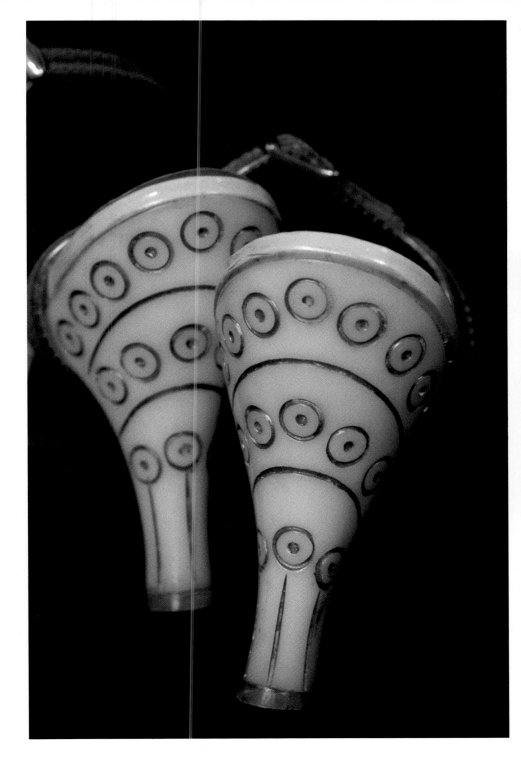

Foot Note on Toes: What do the 1460s and the 1960s have in common? Pointed toes, worn by men and boys. In the 1960s, the "winklepicker" or spike-toed boot was worn by British rockers and their juvenile fans. Due to this exaggerated projection, winklepickers were considered sexual and suggestive. But this had nothing to the *poulaine* that was in fashion five hundred years ago. This was a cloth shoe with a long, tapering toe, clearly phallic. At its zenith, the *poulaine* would reach eighteen inches in length and be padded with horsehair to keep its robust shape. In 1468, a Papal bull denounced the *poulaine* as a lewd and worldly vanity—an edict that was promptly ignored in fashionable circles. The *poulaine* fad waned only when it became so universally popular that the fashion *cognoscenti* at court grew weary of it.

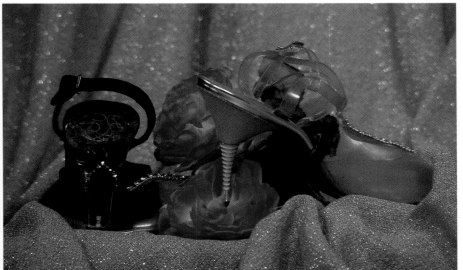

Above: From the late 1950s: rhinestones wrap the heel on black suede sandals by LifeStride, while white-and- silver metal spikes up a pair of "glass slippers" by QualiCraft. *Courtesy of Lindy's Shoppe.* Value: $25-55.

Left: Art deco circles wheel freely on the Bakelite heels of these sandals by Scarpini, circa 1939. *Courtesy of Lindy's Shoppe.* Value: $45-65.

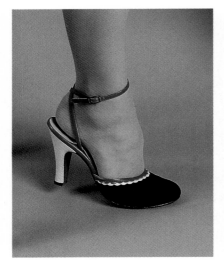

Criss-cross straps serve as heel on a patriotic pump designed by Herbert Levine in the early 1940s, circa 1942. *Collection of Connie Beers*. Value: Special.

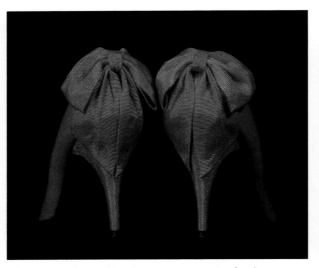

Plump bows form a bustle on a saucy pair of red grosgrain pumps from the mid-1950s, labeled "Park Avenue." *Author's collection*. Value: $15-25.

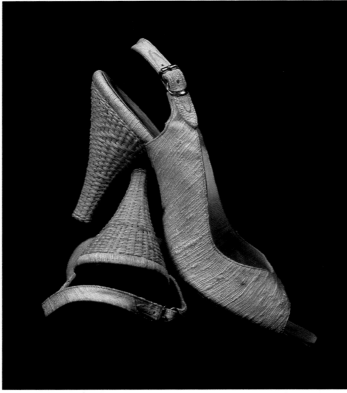

Herbert Levine constructed conical rattan heels for beautiful slingbacks that are wrapped in raw linen, circa 1979. *Courtesy of It's About Time.* Value: $25-45.

Trapunto stitching accents the open toe of spring-green pumps by StylePride, from the early '70s. They are peeping from a decorative Boston Store shoebox, in the vertical shape favored by stylish salons in the 1950s. *Courtesy of Lindy's Shoppe.* Value: shoes, $25-45; box, $10-15.

The Substance

The stuff of which shoes are made is as varied as the imagination of shoe designers. Leather is first, in its various treatments. Then come fabric, wood, metal, rubber, vinyl, cork, and even paper. Sometimes the availability of a new substance is an offshoot of other technologies, such as the breakthrough in vulcanized rubber in the mid-1800s.

Just as often, vanity is the mother of invention, such as the discovery of patent leather in response to a demand for beautiful dance slippers. After all, what better place to pose a dainty foot than at a glittering ball? The dance craze that swept Europe in the eighteenth century created a search by shoemakers for leather with a permanently shiny surface. They first tried a shellac of linseed oil, but this only lent a temporary gloss. In the 1790s, their quest was satisfied by the invention of patent leather.

WE LOVE LEATHER

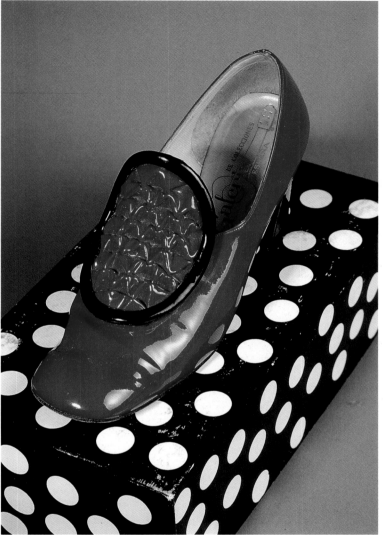

Above: The process of finishing patent leather was developed around 1800, and has been used to good effect in shoe design ever since. The patent sheen looks stiff, which is all the more surprising when it is fashioned like a fine fabric, as in the smocked buckle shown. Also shocking is the bold use of color, reviving a man's brogue style from about 1860 in a low-heeled pump for the gentler sex a full century later. This shoe was imported from Spain under the label Galeria Espana. *Courtesy of Luxe.* Value: $55-65.

Left: Leather is the basic stuff of shoes, sturdy and supple at the same time. Case in point, a pair of basic pumps in fine-grained black kid with a basket weave of leather at the vamp. By the studio label Paramount, circa 1947. *Courtesy of Cheap Thrills.* Value: $25-55.

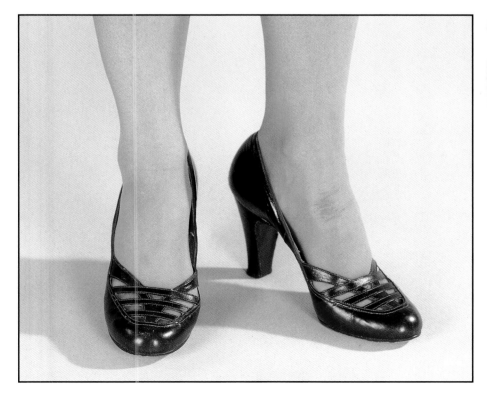

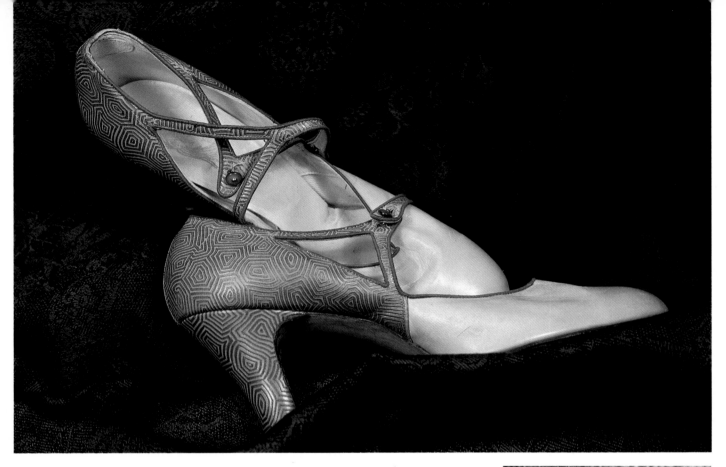

A stylized maze is stamped into fine-grained kid, then dyed
French blue, for the heel and bar of two-tone dress pumps. The
blue mother-of-pearl buttons add a jazzy top note. By Paradise,
they are from the early 1930s as indicated by the slightly rounded
toe. *Collection of Sylvia and Richard Unger.* Value: Special.

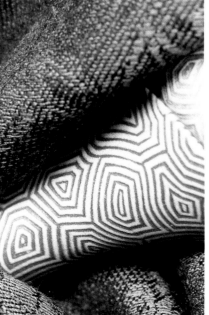

FALL FOR SUEDE

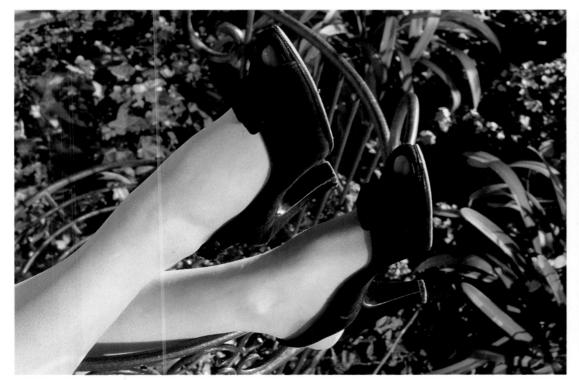

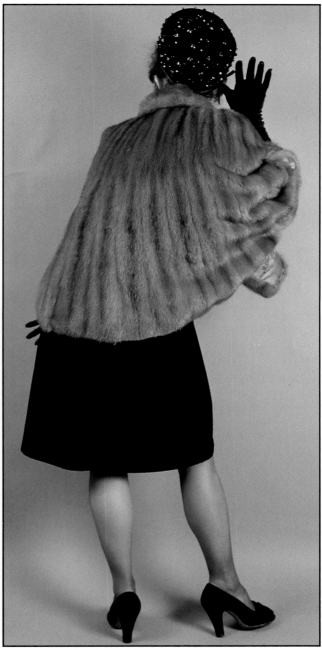

The shoe industry has tried periodically to promote suede for spring, using peep-toes and delicate trim, as in these pumps by Naturalizer, circa 1950. *Courtesy of Cheap Thrills*. Value: $35-55.

Consumers steadfastly wait for the fall and winter to strut their suede. This pair, circa 1950, features a suede blossom just above the peep-toe. *Collection of Connie Beers*. Value: $45-55.

REPTILE REVUE

Right: Creamy cobra oxfords, circa 1925, by Foot Delight. Snakeskin was all the rage in the Jazz Age, with its well-deserved reputation for luxurious and uniquely beautiful footwear. *Courtesy of Lottie Ballou.* Value: $55-75.

Below: The ubiquitous croc platform, circa 1945. This pair is relatively pricey, given the quality of its large grain (from the belly of the beast). Note how well the skins were matched to form an intersecting "V" vamp. From Fenton Footwear for Saks Fifth Avenue. *Courtesy of Luxe.* Value: $75-95.

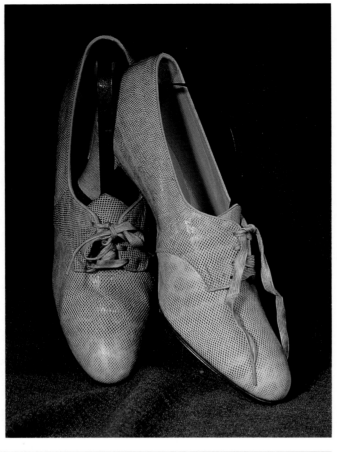

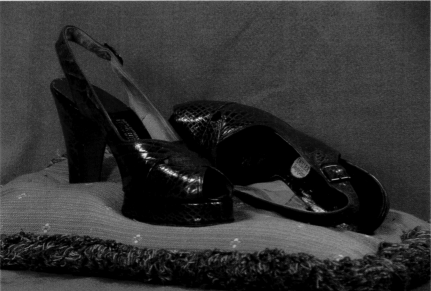

26

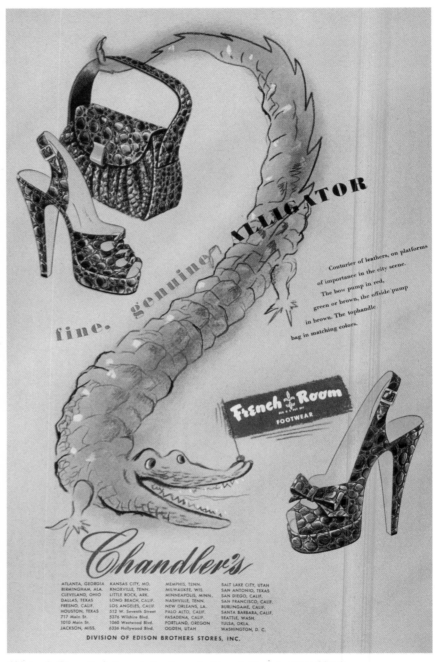

Couturier of leathers, on platforms of importance in the city scene. The bow pump in red, green or brown, the offside pump in brown. The tophandle bag in matching colors.

fine. genuine ALLIGATOR

French Room
FOOTWEAR

Chandler's

ATLANTA, GEORGIA	KANSAS CITY, MO.	MEMPHIS, TENN.	SALT LAKE CITY, UTAH
BIRMINGHAM, ALA.	KNOXVILLE, TENN.	MILWAUKEE, WIS.	SAN ANTONIO, TEXAS
CLEVELAND, OHIO	LITTLE ROCK, ARK.	MINNEAPOLIS, MINN.	SAN DIEGO, CALIF.
DALLAS, TEXAS	LONG BEACH, CALIF.	NASHVILLE, TENN.	SAN FRANCISCO, CALIF.
FRESNO, CALIF.	LOS ANGELES, CALIF.	NEW ORLEANS, LA.	BURLINGAME, CALIF.
HOUSTON, TEXAS	512 W. Seventh Street	PALO ALTO, CALIF.	SANTA BARBARA, CALIF.
717 Main St.	5376 Wilshire Blvd.	PASADENA, CALIF.	SEATTLE, WASH.
1010 Main St.	1060 Westwood Blvd.	PORTLAND, OREGON	TULSA, OKLA.
JACKSON, MISS.	6336 Hollywood Blvd.	OGDEN, UTAH	WASHINGTON, D. C.

DIVISION OF EDISON BROTHERS STORES, INC.

Although Chandler's is a chain store, its French Room carried high-quality footwear in the 1930s, '40s, and '50s. This advertisement shows alligator "platforms of importance in the city scene." The bow pump came in red, green, or brown; the bag was dyed-to-match.

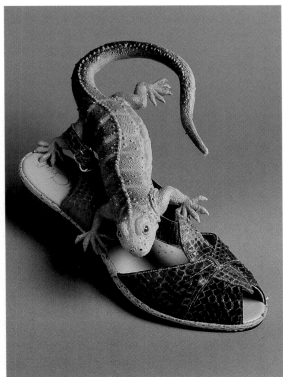

Since the early 1920s, reptile has been died in brilliant shades of red, violet, ochre, and green. At first this type of workmanship was reserved for custom-made shoes. This charming color palette soon spread to mass production, as in these sunny sandals from the mid-1940s. *Courtesy of Luxe.* Value: $45-65.

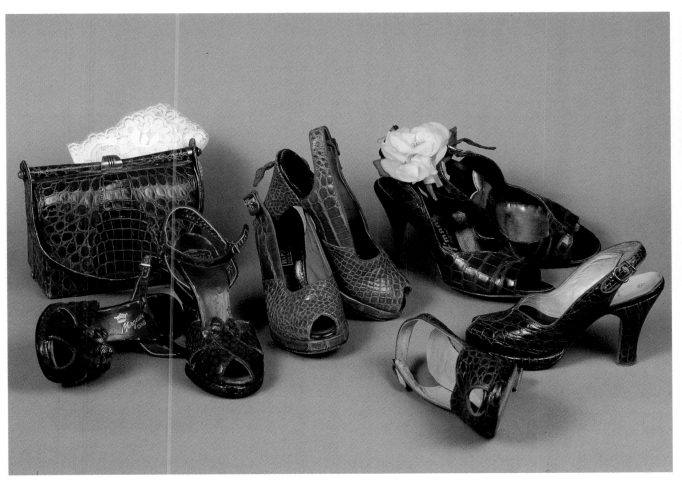

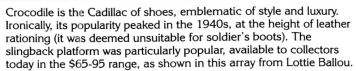

Crocodile is the Cadillac of shoes, emblematic of style and luxury. Ironically, its popularity peaked in the 1940s, at the height of leather rationing (it was deemed unsuitable for soldier's boots). The slingback platform was particularly popular, available to collectors today in the $65-95 range, as shown in this array from Lottie Ballou.

A METAL URGE

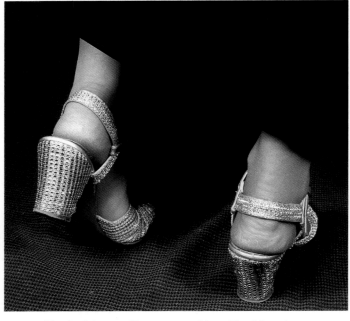

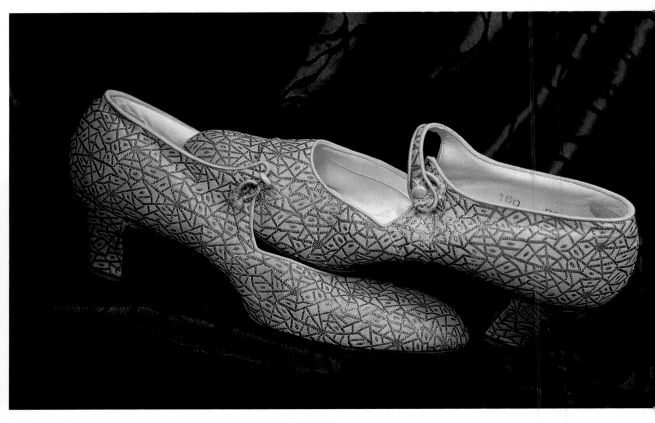

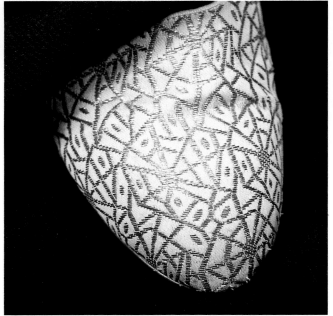

The look is metallic weave, achieved by thin strips of gold and silver celluloid. These are from the late 1930s and feature the chunky heel so popular then. *Courtesy of Lottie Ballou.* Value: $15-35.

Above & Left: Single-bar pumps cut from an amazing jacquard, a spider web design woven in silver thread on a background of cream chain stitch. Despite signs of heavy wear on the soles of these shoes, the uppers appear near-new—evidence that this seemingly fragile fabric has the tensile strength of steel! The shoes were made by A.M. Williams & Co. in the late 1920s. *Courtesy of Sylvia and Richard Unger.* Value: Special.

28

Holding On

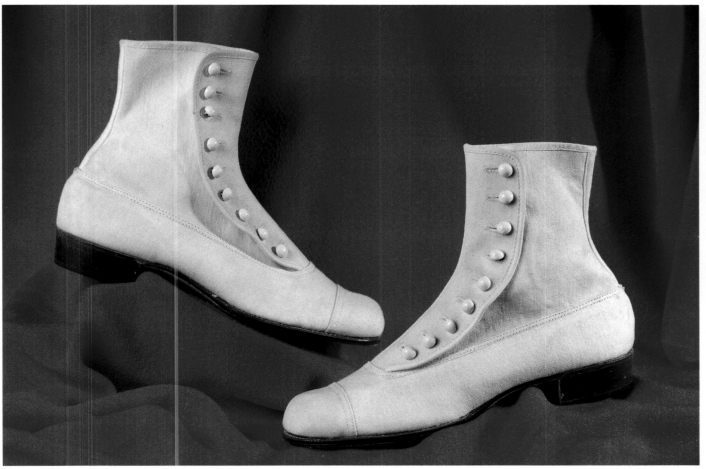

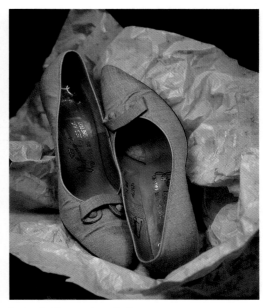

Later in the century, buttons were merely decorative. The button-and-tab device at the toe of these linen pumps was also a popular motif for suit jackets, circa 1955. The label is Johnny's Hand-Made. *Courtesy of It's About Time.* Value: $15-25.

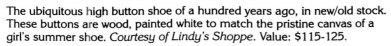

The ubiquitous high button shoe of a hundred years ago, in new/old stock. These buttons are wood, painted white to match the pristine canvas of a girl's summer shoe. *Courtesy of Lindy's Shoppe.* Value: $115-125.

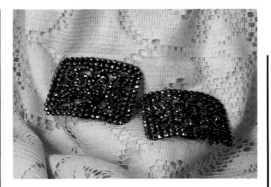

Since the days of Queen Victoria, women have used removable buckles to dress up plain pumps at a relatively low cost. The cut steel version is circa 1915 while the sweet blue rhinestone bows are circa 1955. *Courtesy of Rich Man, Poor Man.* Value: $35-55.

Silver buckles are reflected in silver heels, as a functional element of design. These sandals were imported from Italy in the early 1970s. They are modeled by Barbara Grigg, owner of a vintage clothing business in Lafayette, California. "I must have a good eye for shoes, because I certainly can't keep them in my own closet for long. My friends are always buying them from me." Indeed, it is Barbara who supplied many of the other Bay Area collectors who generously loaned shoes for the photographs in this book.

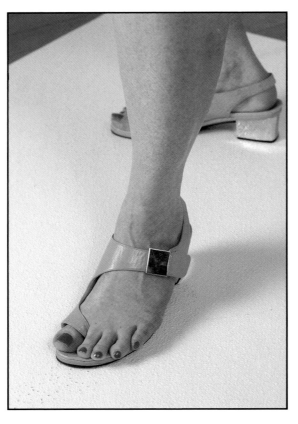

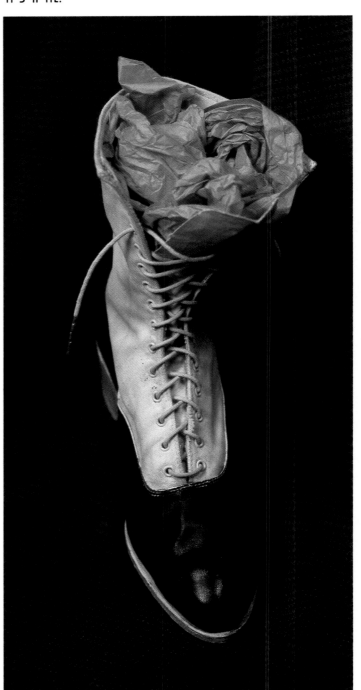

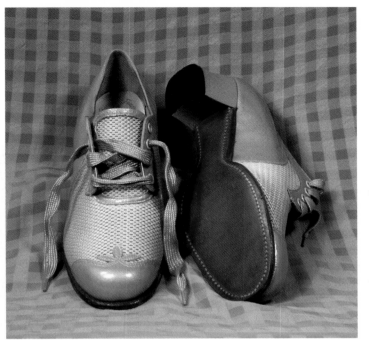

The classic laced-up oxford in new\old stock from the 1920s in a relatively unusual size 10B. Note the delicate leaf detail where pearl green leather meets creamy cotton mesh. These are the Tryle Walk label by Miller of Sacramento. *Courtesy of Gail Pocock.* Value: $75-95.

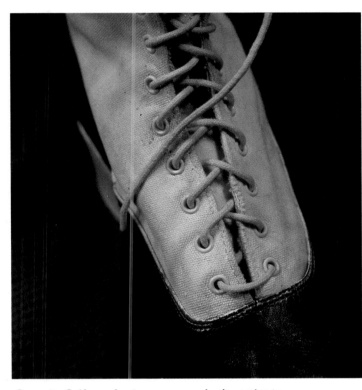

Opposite & Above: Lacing was an early alternative to shoe buttons, having made an appearance at the ankle of low booties in the mid-1800s. By the turn-of-the-century, high boots were laced up the front, typically with leather or cotton cord. This is an early spectator, sporty in black patent and white canvas. The stacked wooden heel was painted white by a later owner. *Courtesy of It's About Time.* Value: $75-95 for the pair.

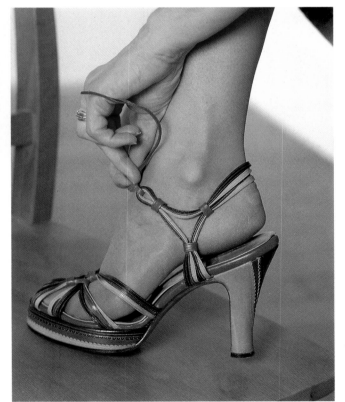

Sandals don't get more strippy-strappy than this, in tri-tone leather platforms. Circa 1975, from the Hertz-Ross shoe salon in Miami Beach. *Courtesy of Luxe.* Value: $55-75.

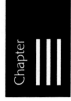

Chapter III

WITH PASSION

Shoes have always been charged with significant sexual connotation. Chinese foot-binding was an extreme example, when the deformed foot became an object of erotic desire. No less so, the tightly laced boots of fetishism, which promise a release of passion, along with that of the bound flesh.

Not all passion associated with a woman's shoe is carnal. Shoes are also a symbol of romantic love and a token of fidelity. In the peasant societies of sixteenth century Europe, a young man would give shoes to show his lass that he wanted to share his worldly goods with her. During the late eighteenth century, it was all the rage among romantics of the British upper crust to troth their love with the gift of a delicate porcelain slipper. Later, the sentimental Victorians exchanged miniature shoes of glass, china, velvet, wood, and metal as a courtship ritual.

Of course, the Victorians were not always sentimental—they could also be naughty. Vintage fashion collectors may be familiar with the use of corsets as a motif for cufflinks and cigar cutters. Translated into shoe lore, the trait turned up in curious renderings of high heels and laced boots on flasks, snuffboxes, and cane handles.

The Sexy Shoe

When a woman crosses her legs to dangle a high heel; or shifts in her chair to fuss with an ankle strap; or strolls from a dance floor with sandals slung over her shoulder, she is publicly signaling sexual availability. Some shoes are so intrinsically sexy, that flirtatious gestures with the foot would be redundant. In France, an ornamental heel is called *venez y vair*, which roughly translates as "come-hither."

In 1984, the venerable *Wall Street Journal* reported on shoe design in decidedly racy terms: "The pump (has) a low-cut look in the so-called throat line, which means the shoe shows more of the cracks between the toes. The industry calls this 'cleavage.' "

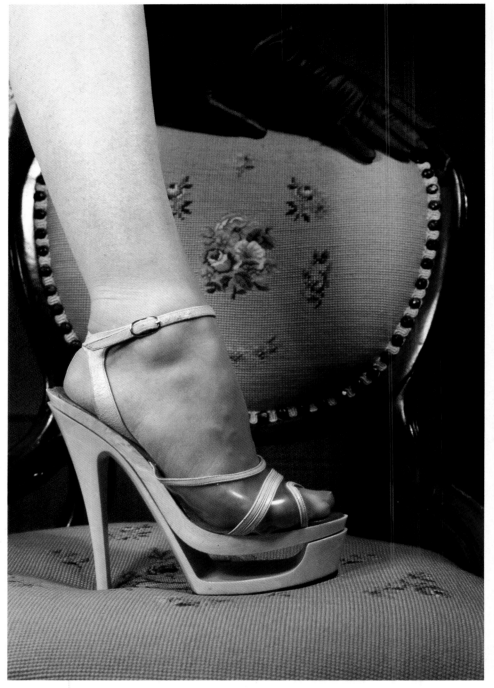

These Italian imports are from the Sexy Sixties in molded plastic and vinyl, and are aptly labeled The Wild Pair. They walk a fine line between funk and fetish on towering wedge *cum* stiletto heels that tip the tape measure at 5.5 inches. *Collection of Rhonda Barrett.* Value: $55-75.

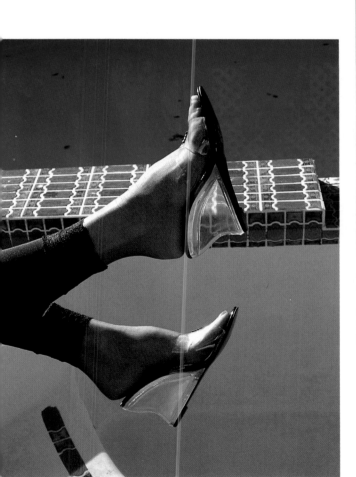

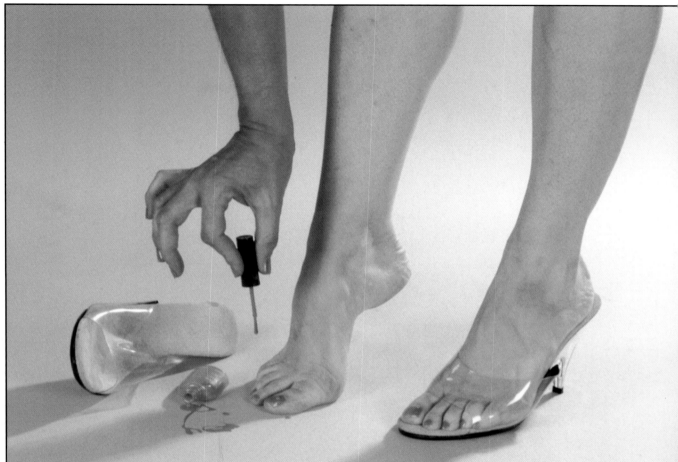

Above: Cinderella gets sexy in a "glass" slipper, circa 1975. *Courtesy of Cheap Thrills.* Value: $15-35.

Left: The vinyl vamp, the Lucite wedgie. The label Syvel's Classics is justified since this glitzy style has been popular from the '40s to the present day. *Author's collection.* Value: $15-35.

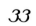

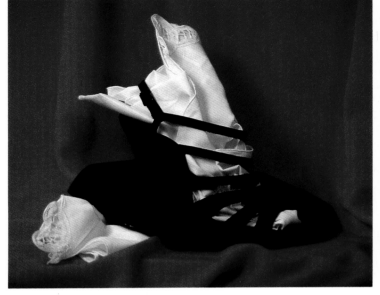

The black plate special. One order of strappy black sandals from Marshall Field & Co., circa 1960. *Courtesy of Luxe.* Value: $35-55.

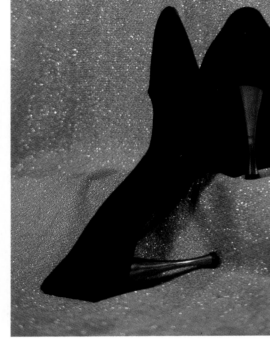

Stilettos were the very height of style in 1967. These black suede shoes with gold spike heels were designed by Julianelli some 30 years ago. *Courtesy of Barbara Grigg Vintage Fashion.* Value: $75-95.

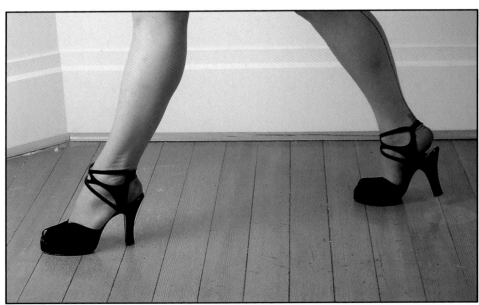

What a web of intrigue you will weave wearing "Spider Woman" ankle straps circa 1945. Custom-crafted by Lindburg's of Oakland. *Collection of Connie Beers*. Value: Special.

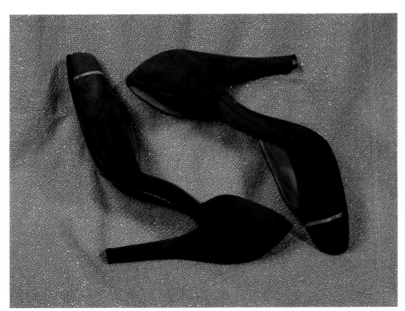

Brown suede is cut daringly low, on four-inch heels up to no good. These brazen beauties from the mid-1960s are by Norman Kaplan. *Author's collection*. Value: $55-75.

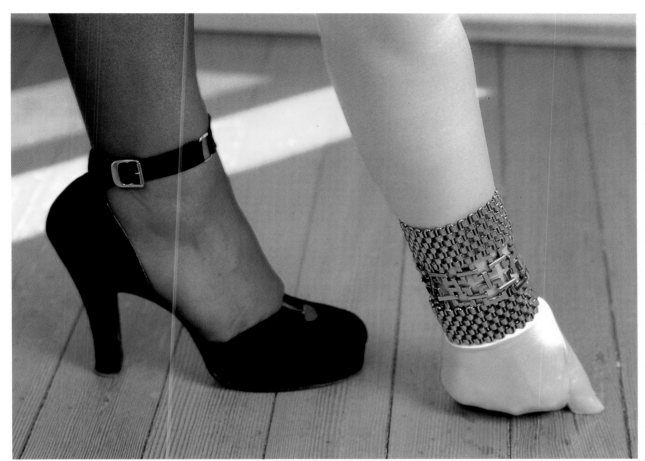

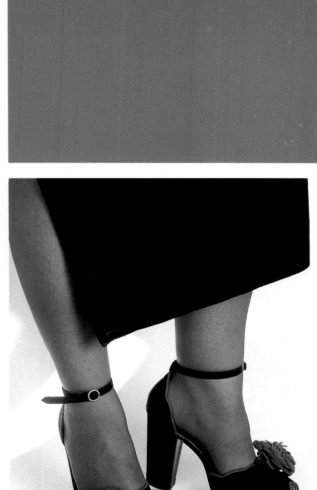

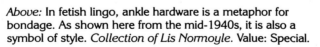

Above: In fetish lingo, ankle hardware is a metaphor for bondage. As shown here from the mid-1940s, it is also a symbol of style. *Collection of Lis Normoyle.* Value: Special.

Right: Lis Normoyle bought these black suede platforms by Chelsea Cobblers in London. "It was 1972, and even then they cost me 45 pounds. That was half the expense money I'd brought with me, but I just had to have them! I would dance all night in these—amazing I didn't break an ankle." Indeed. Lis had good reason to love shoes, having just opened a boutique in Southern California catering to the "hippie chic" crowd. Now she sells luxury vintage clothing to an upscale clientele from her shop *Luxe,* in Palo Alto, California.

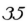

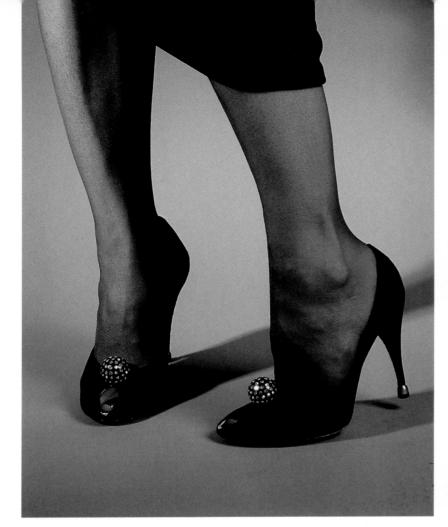

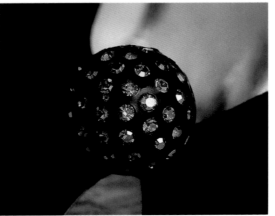

The *diamonté* ball made famous as a heel by Roger Vivier moves to the toe of these pumps, circa 1985, from the house label Christian Dior. *Courtesy of Luxe.* Value: $75-95.

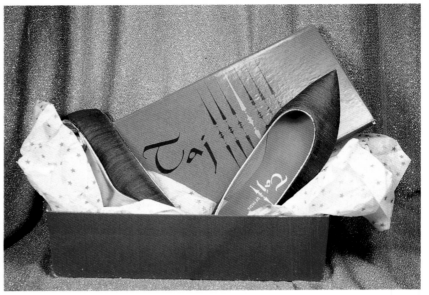

In the late 1950s, Taj Tajerie designed his signature gold-soled Ottoman slipper for Gloria Swanson, and glamorous ladies everywhere. These sexy flats shown were never worn and are shown in the original box. Not one to hide his light under a minaret, Tajerie included a card in each box proclaiming: "East meets West in this luxurious special-occasion shoe (with) the shape of India in the traditional upturned toe . . . the opulence of India in the golden soles and heels (and) . . . the inspired know-how of a famous designer." *Author's collection.* Value: $25-45.

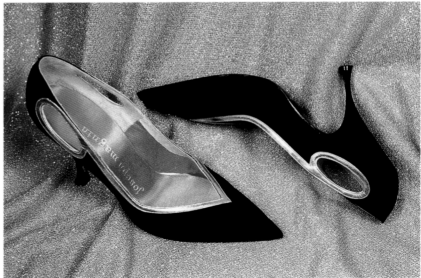

Thanks to her impeccable lineage from the design talent of Herbert Levine, this 1970s shoe is quite the lady, despite her décolleté vamp and peek-a-boo heel. In black silk with gold kid, and the surprise of fuchsia satin lining. *Author's collection.* Value: $45-65.

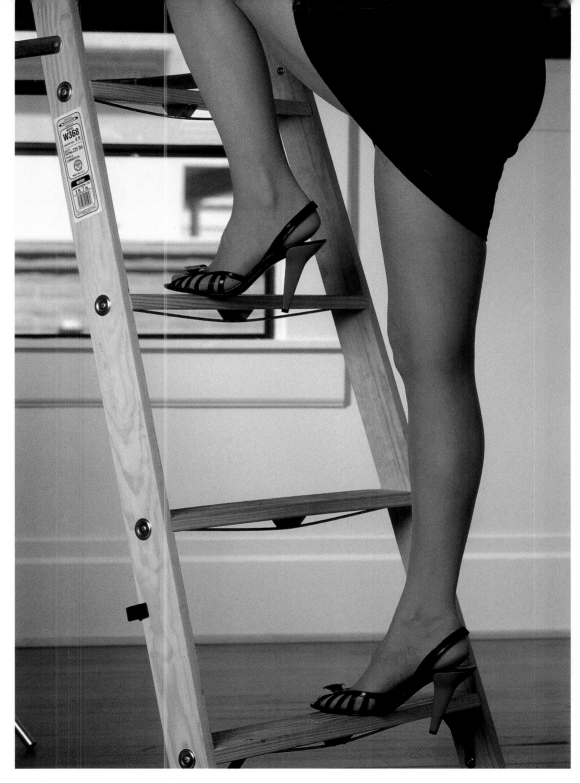

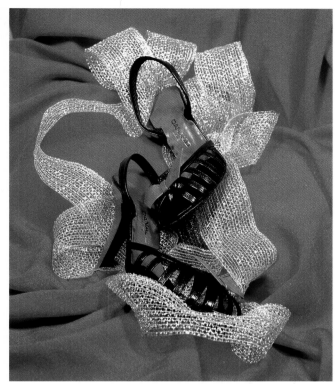

Left & Above: Women will go to great heights for an alluring pair of legs, as the French have always known. Note the saucy pink bows on the toes of these spike heels by Xavier Danaud, Paris. *Collection of Lis Normoyle.* Value: Special.

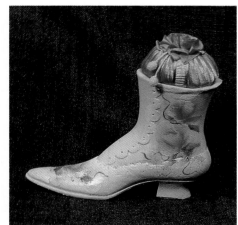

This charming high-button shoe was cast from an antique mold, then hand-painted by artisan Viola De Cou. The Victorian original was the type exchanged between sweethearts, as a symbol of fidelity and a token of affection.

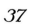

Still the Stiletto

In the seventeenth century, the British Parliament passed a law making it grounds for divorce if a man testified that he was tricked into marriage by a woman wearing high heels.

To balance in heels, a woman must thrust her chest forward and reduce her steps from stride to mince. With her pelvis at a tilt, she will also sway from side-to-side with an undulating motion. The allure is primal, and unmistakable. Or, as sexologist Alfred Kinsey observed, when a woman is aroused she arches her foot until it "falls in line with the rest of the leg." Sounds like high heels!

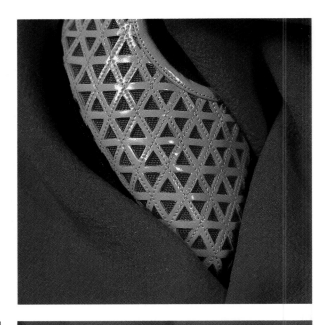

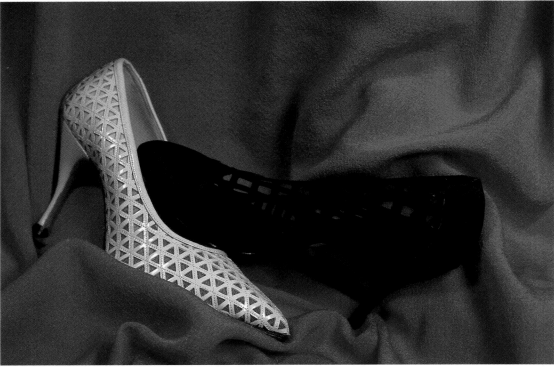

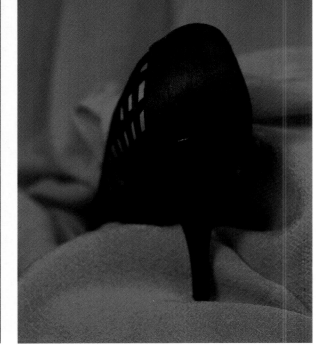

These meticulous mesh pumps were machine-stitched in cream patent leather by Delman, and in black silk by Herbert Levine. The pointy-toe stiletto was *the* shoe silhouette of the early 1960s. *Courtesy of It's About Time.* Value: $25-45.

"Stilettos are about sex, and what I mean by that is that female baboons, when they're aroused, walk on their tiptoes. It's a true fact."
—Tom Ford, for Gucci.

"Learning to walk in high heels is like learning to ride a bicycle. Practice, practice, practice! But don't think too much about pitfalls. When a woman wears high heels, there are only three real, hopefully insurmountable pitfalls—men, men, men."
—Manolo Blahnik, 1997, at the height of a revival in high heels that he helped to create

"If you rebel against high-heeled shoes, take care to do so in a very smart hat."
—British playwright George Bernard Shaw

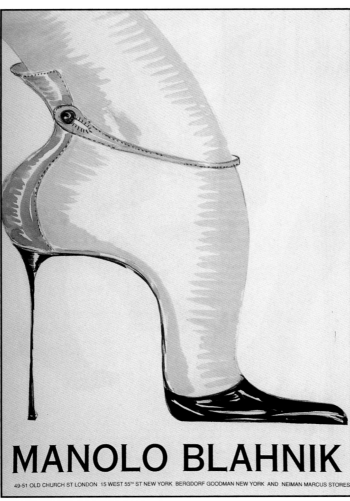

MANOLO BLAHNIK

49-51 OLD CHURCH ST LONDON 15 WEST 55TH ST NEW YORK BERGDORF GOODMAN NEW YORK AND NEIMAN MARCUS STORES

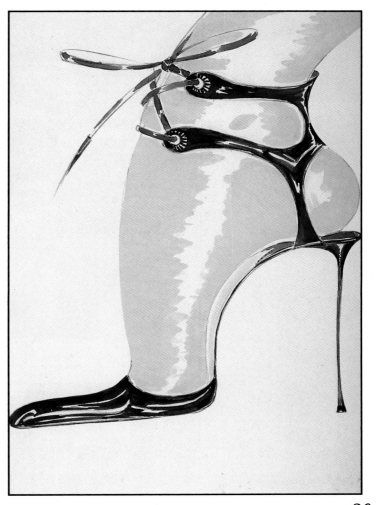

Manolo Blahnik was one of many top-flight designers who revived the stiletto in 1997, with an edgy new attitude.

39

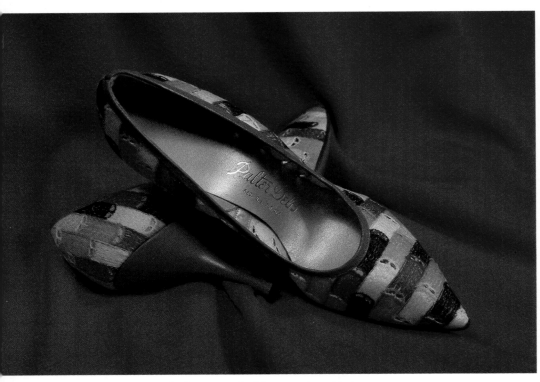

An amazing pair of stilettos, crafted from custom fabric by Palter De Liso for his Palter Debs line. The silk is textured like bark and spun into three shades of tan shingles. *Courtesy of It's About Time.* Value: $35-55.

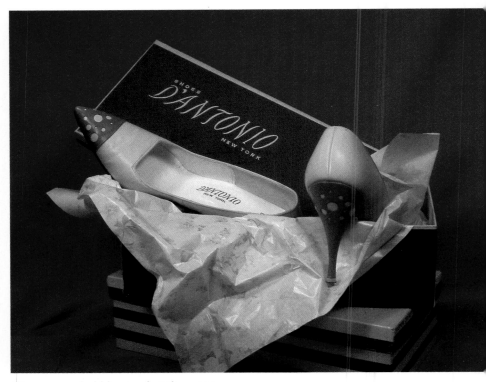

Champagne bubbles on absinthe-green leather, a fine example of the pointy-toe stiletto. Imported from Italy by D'Antonio. *Courtesy of It's About Time.* Value: $25-45.

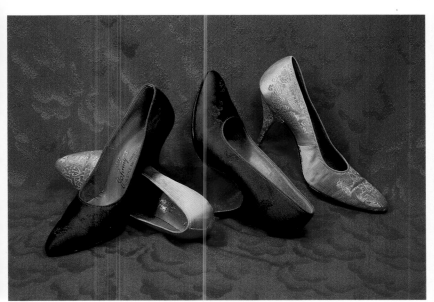

The stiletto in teal silk and ivory silk jacquard.
Note the oriental design of the jacquard, which
was all the rage in the mid-1960s. Both pairs of
pumps are labeled "Handmade by Johnny."
Courtesy of It's About Time. Value: $25-45.

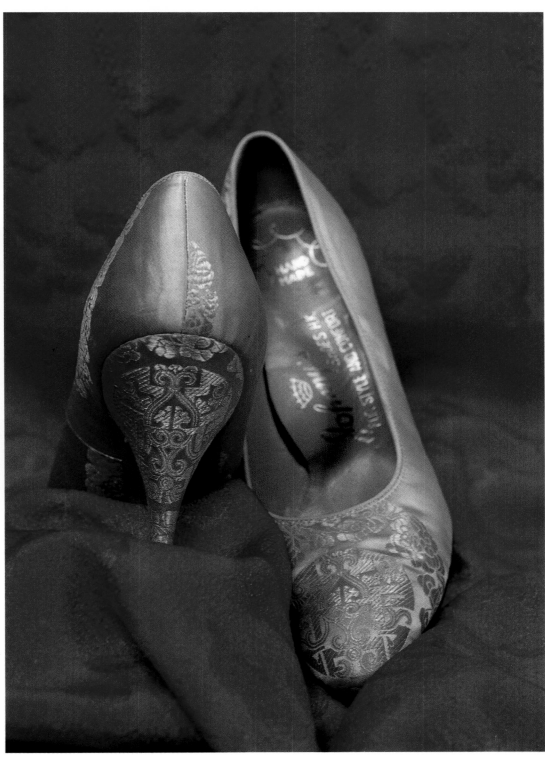

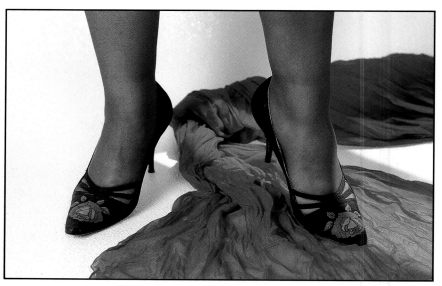

One perfect red rose blooms forever on a silk-screened party pump by Qualicraft. *Courtesy of Luxe.* Value: $25-45.

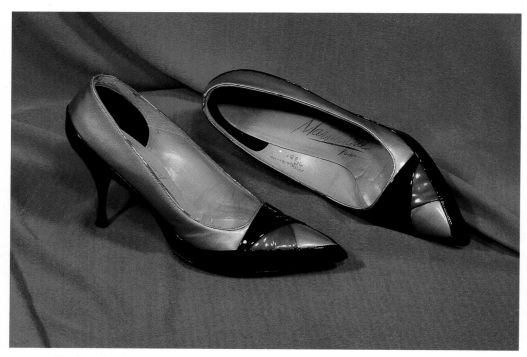

Vinylized leather in a patriotic tri-tone by Martinique. *Courtesy of Rich Man, Poor Man.* Value: $15-25.

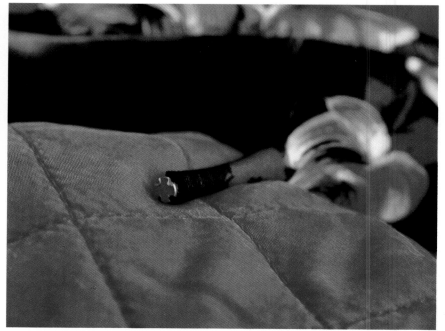

Up close and personal, the steel core of a stiletto heel. This is the nail-like tip that caused so much damage to wooden floors that it was banned from certain public buildings during the 1960s.

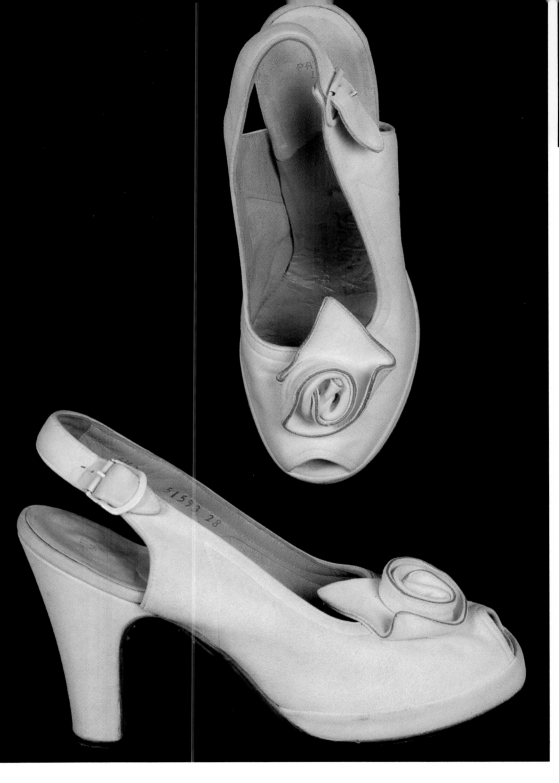

IV OR IS IT ART?

Shoe as Sculpture

"Shoe design is a sculptural problem in which the center is always a void."
—Roger Vivier.

Petals of sueded white leather unfurl, sweet with the promise of eternal spring. These mid-1940s slingback platforms were designed by Palter DeLiso. *Courtesy of Lottie Ballou.* Value: $75-95.

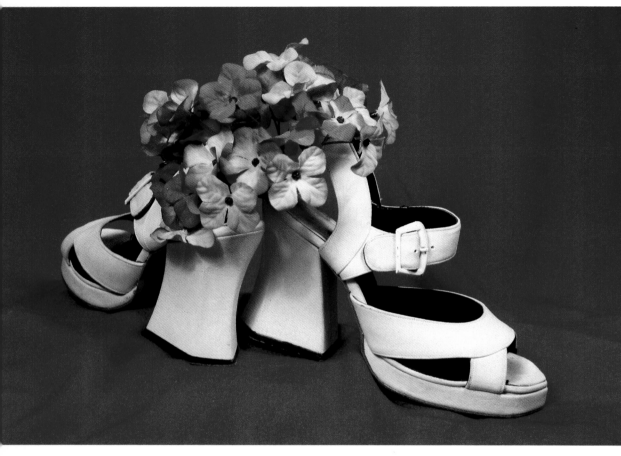

Scoops of white suede create linear tension with a curvilinear tease. Note the painted metal buckle on these pre-war platforms from Buffums of California. *Courtesy of Luxe.* Value: $95-115.

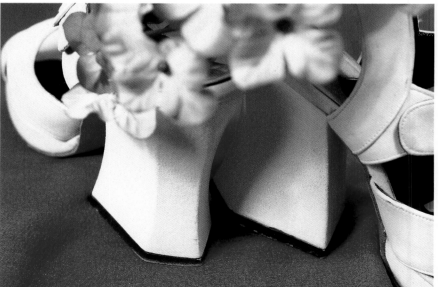

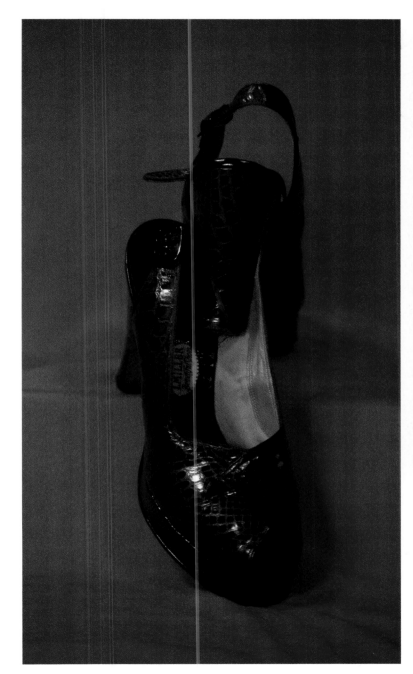

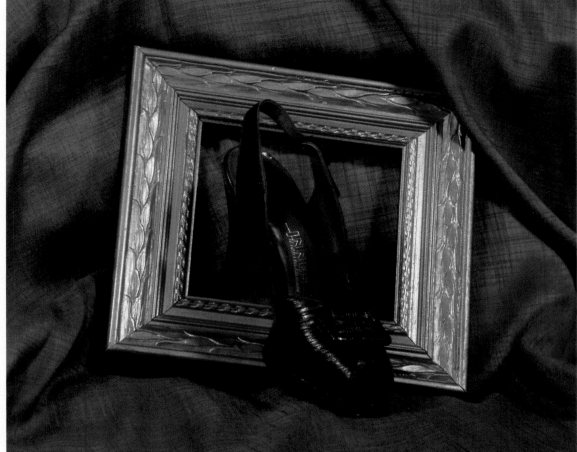

Above: Steppin' out in steel gray lizard slingback platforms. The label is LizaGator, sold at I. Miller in the late 1940s. *Courtesy of Lindy's Shoppe.* Value: $35-55.

Left: If you could only own one pair of alligator shoes, let it be these. Gleaming mahogany patterned to perfection, from the mid-1940s. *Courtesy of Luxe.* Value: $75-95.

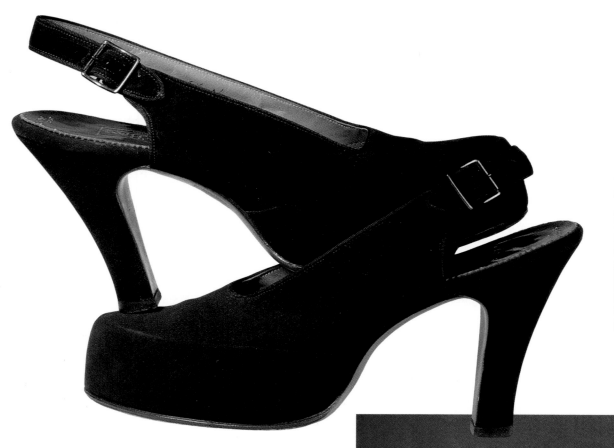

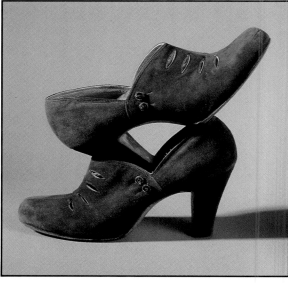

Dance the jig in these emerald suede Leprechaun shoes from Harzfeld's in Kansas City, circa 1935. *Courtesy of Lottie Ballou.* Value: $65-85.

Platforms make a hot silhouette in coffee suede, circa 1945. *Courtesy of Lottie Ballou.* Value: $95-115.

A zigzag ziggurat in pewter leather glows against soft gray suede, the only ornament on half-inch high platforms. This motif references the earlier Art Deco movement, from an unknown designer in the mid-1940s. *Courtesy of Past Perfect.* Value: $95-115.

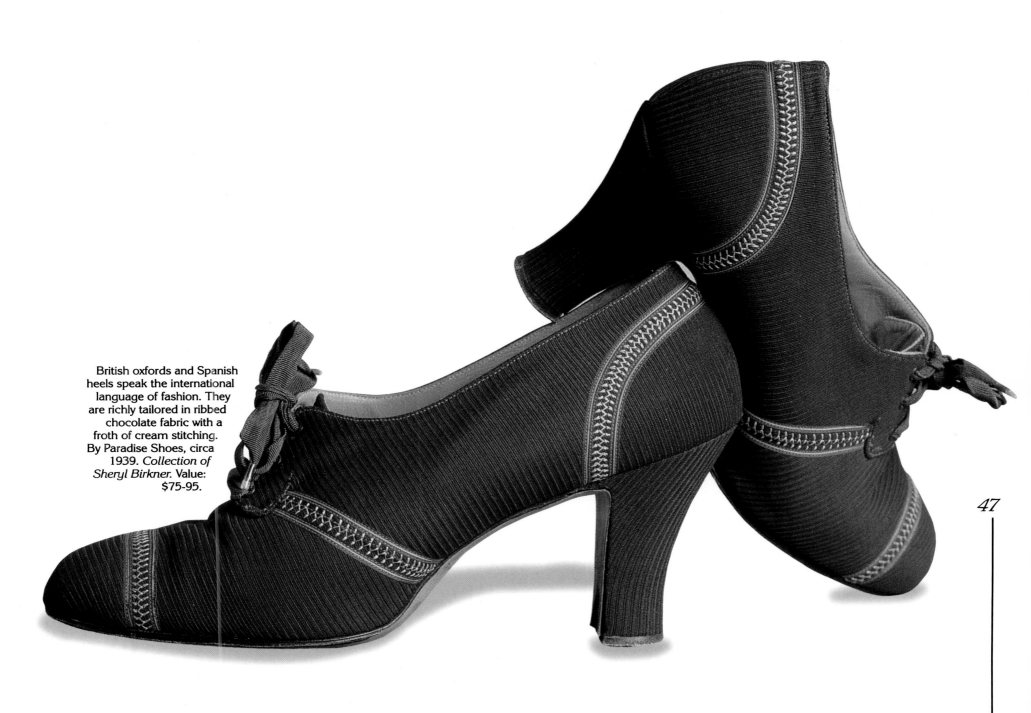

British oxfords and Spanish heels speak the international language of fashion. They are richly tailored in ribbed chocolate fabric with a froth of cream stitching. By Paradise Shoes, circa 1939. *Collection of Sheryl Birkner.* Value: $75-95.

47

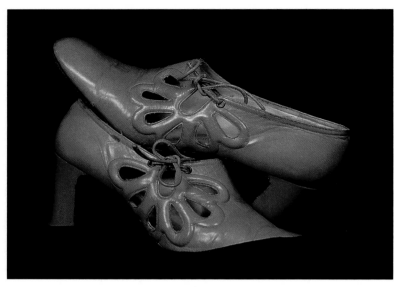

The petal-shape was popular in the 1960s. It's shown here outlined in topstitching on fine leather boot shoes imported from Italy. *Courtesy of It's About Time.* Value: $25-45.

Its fashion fusion with an edge, when passionate straps meet ice-sculpture heel. These ankle-wrap sandals are by Lady McGuire, circa 1975. *Courtesy of It's About Time.* Value: $35-55.

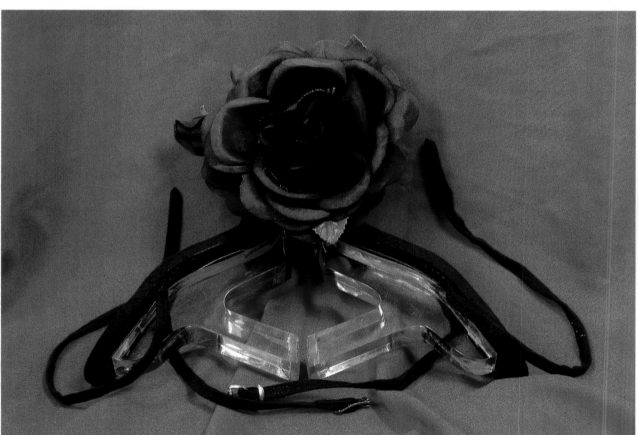

On a Pedestal

It takes a while to adjust the eye to sudden shifts in fashion. When Vivier sketched his first raft platform sandal in 1937, it was too radical for Herman Delman, for whom he usually designed. Not so for Elsa Schiaparelli, who saw the shoe with an artist's eye (and a surrealist one, at that). She commissioned the style for her next collection, and the rest is shoe history.

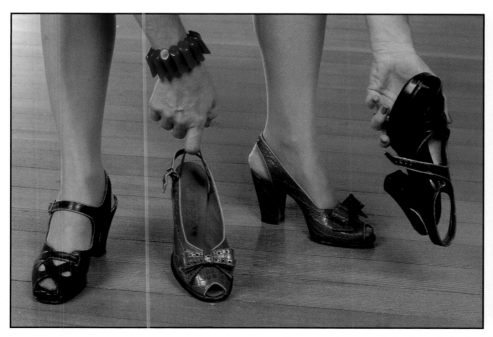

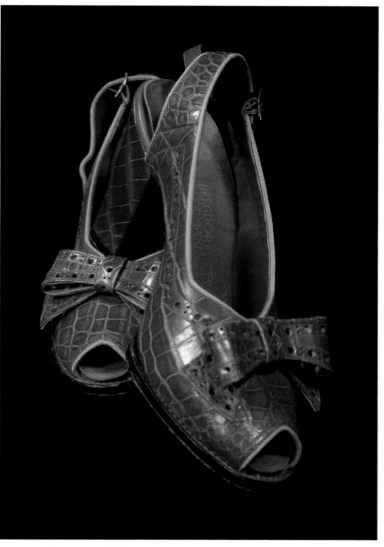

So many shoes, so little time. Debating the merits of open-toe platforms from the mid-1940s, in duotone kid and red crocodile. She prefers the red with its perky bow-tie by Delman for the shoe salon at Bergdorf Goodman's. *Duotone courtesy of Lottie Ballou; red from author's collection.* Value: $65-85.

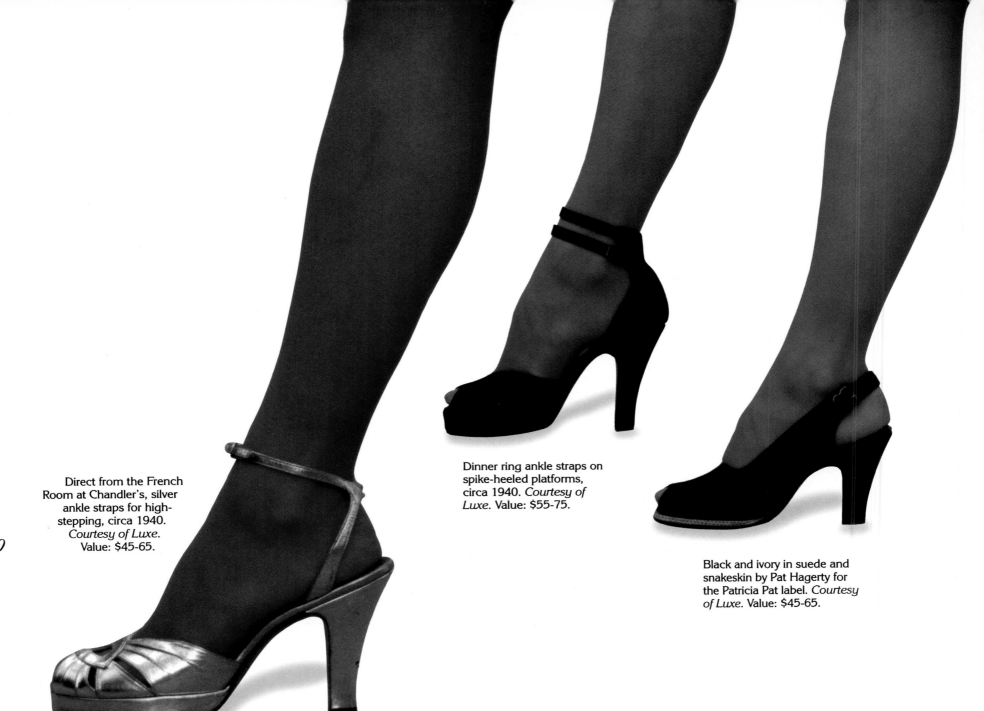

Direct from the French Room at Chandler's, silver ankle straps for high-stepping, circa 1940. *Courtesy of Luxe.* Value: $45-65.

50

Dinner ring ankle straps on spike-heeled platforms, circa 1940. *Courtesy of Luxe.* Value: $55-75.

Black and ivory in suede and snakeskin by Pat Hagerty for the Patricia Pat label. *Courtesy of Luxe.* Value: $45-65.

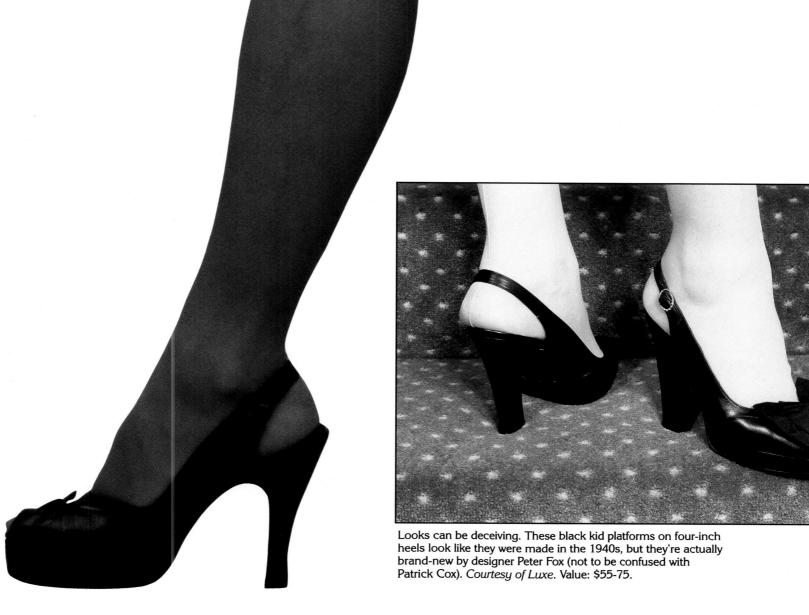

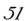

The cut-out vamp is a nice touch in dark coffee suede, from Beleganti, circa 1949. *Courtesy of Luxe.* Value: $55-75.

Looks can be deceiving. These black kid platforms on four-inch heels look like they were made in the 1940s, but they're actually brand-new by designer Peter Fox (not to be confused with Patrick Cox). *Courtesy of Luxe.* Value: $55-75.

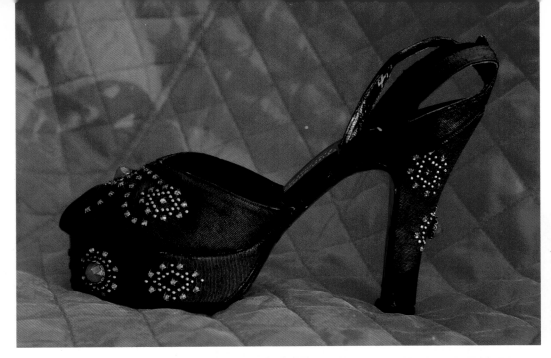

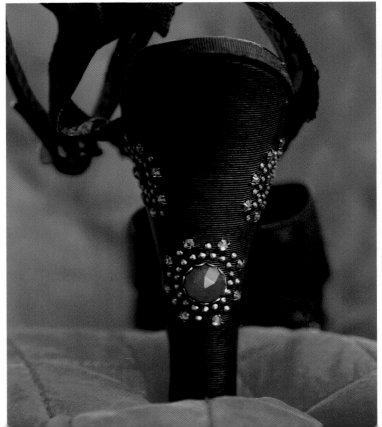

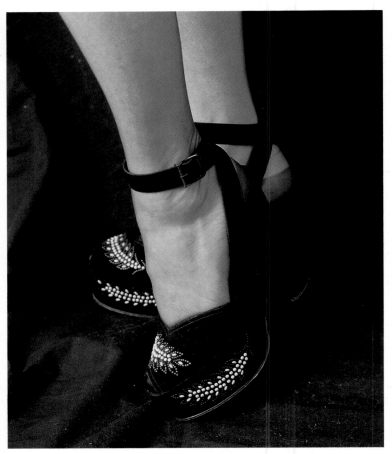

Above & Right: A traffic-stopping platform in black grosgrain, with "rubies" the size of headlights. By the Metro Shoe Co., circa 1948. *Author's collection.* Value: $75-95.

Fabulous faux turquoise stones are scattered around black suede platforms by Morris Wolock. These higher soles were worn in the mid- and late-1940s. *Collection of Pamela Joyce.* Value: Special.

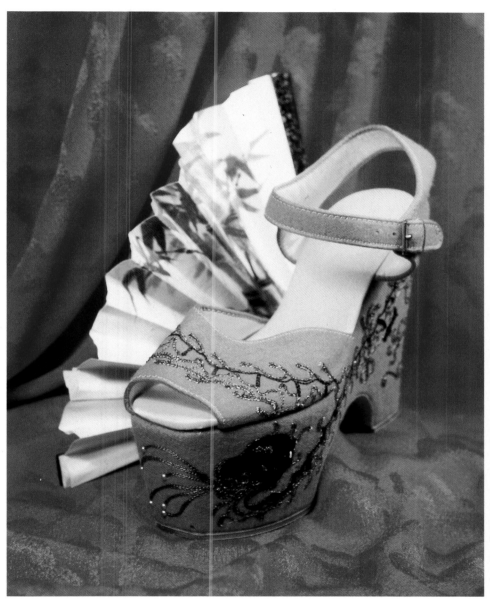

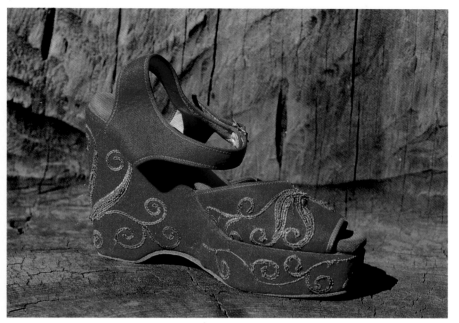

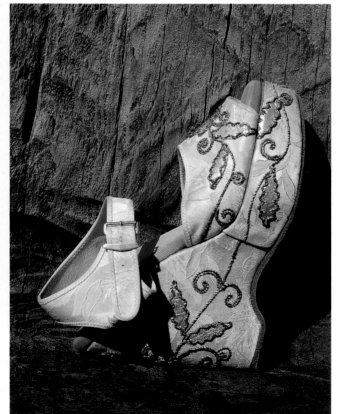

Above & Left: Two more rafts, strikingly similar to the dragon-lady pair. Again, the uppers are felted wool and the trim is unusual, most likely the result of wartime shortages. The white platforms are accented with silver-kid leaves; the red relies on gilt cording. *Courtesy of Deco Diva.* Value: $55-75.

The shoe designer is unknown, but this platform sandal owes a lot to Schiaparelli's raft design of 1938 (which was itself attributed to Vivier). Of interest, the cowhide soles are stamped "Patent Applied For." Note the innovative mix of materials, with uppers of felted wool and a lining of rayon. The fiery dragon is formed by machine chain-stitch with gold ball accents. *Collection of Marcia del Toro.* Value: Special.

Deco Delight

Throughout the 1920s and in the years that followed World War I, there was a real renaissance in the craft of shoe manufacture. This was partly due to new technical developments and the refined use of aniline dyes.

It was also attributable to the increasingly active role of women outside the home. Having worked in munitions plants and field hospitals, women were ready for freedom of movement. The dress reform dream of the suffragettes was finally to become reality for the common woman. This meant shorter skirts and a spotlight on shoes!

It was not long after the first World War that the world experienced an explosion in the arts, both fine and applied. The motif of machinery and the streamlining of style became a hallmark of the 1925 Paris *Exposition Internationale des Arts Decoratifs et Industriels Moderne*. This shoe would define the two great artistic movements that shaped early twentieth century aesthetics: art deco and *moderne*.

The *moderne* eye was applied to all aspects of personal apparel, including footwear. There were new styles, and plenty of them. Materials included fine glove-kid leathers with hand-stitched trim or hand-painted motifs, luxury reptile skins dyed in vivid colors, sleek satin or silk loomed as a complex jacquard with metallic threads, and complex buttons and buckles in mother-of-pearl, strass, bakelite, enamel, and *guilloche*.

It was a prosperous time for many Americans, and many could afford to purchase multiple pairs of shoes each season. Yet the cost of labor and services, dependent on the burgeoning immigrant population, was relatively cheap. Many of the finer shoe stores would custom fit their regular clientele, or make shoes to order.

The Great Depression of 1929 abruptly ended casual luxuries for all but the very wealthy. Perversely, the depression created a quest for quality goods that could be depended upon to last. The overall emphasis was on classic styling, with a strong influence of art deco still evident in buckles, buttons, and other trim. Removable buckles were popular because they could give several new looks to the same basic pair of pumps.

Women's shoes of the art deco era are a delight for the collector. They are varied, stylish, amusing, classic, graceful, and sensual—a combination of craft and art that left a legacy of excellence in design.

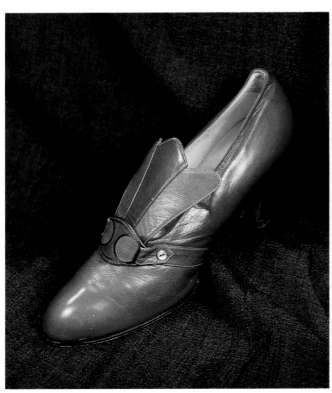

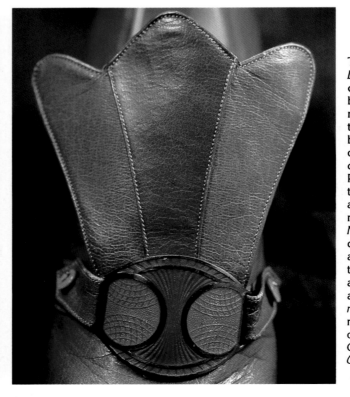

These shoes speak the language of *Les Arts Decoratif*. The stunning contrast of jade green and French blue kid is typical of the early to mid-1920s. Note the machine-turning effect in the cloisonné buckle, and the stylized fan-shape of the tongue. By an unknown designer, perhaps inspired by Perugia. Sylvia Unger acquired these museum-quality shoes from a friend, who had worn them in a national dress competition for Model-T car clubs. "I begged her, don't ever sell these shoes to anyone but me! No one could give them a better home." Suitably, she and her husband Richard—also an avid collector—live in an *art moderne* flat. They are active members of the Art Deco Society of California in Sacramento. *Collection of Sylvia and Richard Unger.* Value, the pair: Special.

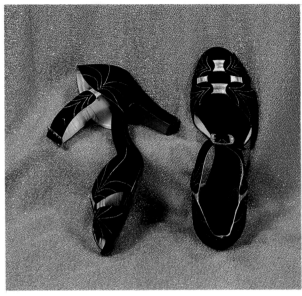

Black silk trimmed with gold and silver kid on dance shoes from the early 1930s. The talented designer is unknown, but may have hailed from San Francisco. An identical pair of mint-condition shoes were featured in a recent exhibition by the De Young Museum in that city. *Courtesy of Lottie Ballou.* Value: $75-95.

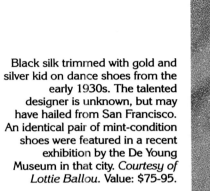

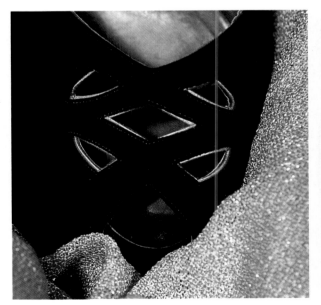

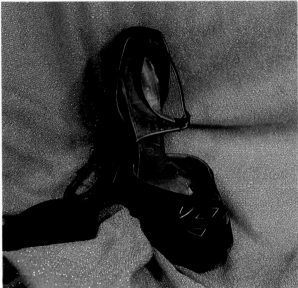

Gold-rimmed diamonds fit for the silver screen, by Sydney of Hollywood, circa 1945. *Collection of Connie Beers.* Value: Special.

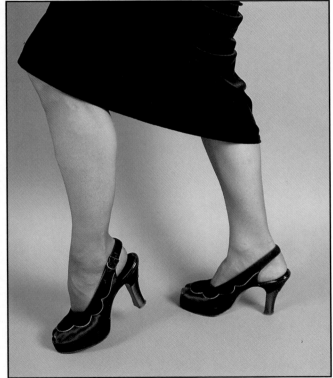

These black suede platforms feature satin scallops outlined in gold braid. For a night of Hollywood glamour by Mackey Starr, designer to the stars, circa 1948. *Collection of Connie Birkner.* Value: Special.

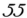

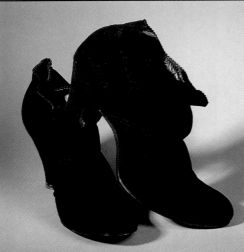

Left: Ruffled ankle boots, with just a hint of court jester. The medieval look was briefly popular in the late 1930s and early '40s (when ruffled and parti-colored suede ankle boots were shown by Perugia). These stunners are by Bally under the label Importe de Suisse, *Bally's Rouge. Courtesy of Barbara Grigg Vintage Fashion.* Value: $125-145.

Below: Dial "D" for Deco. High-vamp shoes in black suede, well-paired with a telephone purse, both circa 1935. (Look closely to see the designer label on the phone dial: "Anne Maris, 228 Rue de Rivoli, Hotel Meurice, Paris." Shoe label is unknown.) *Shoes courtesy of Barbara Grigg Vintage Fashion; bag courtesy of Luxe.* Value: shoes, $75-95; bag, $95-115.

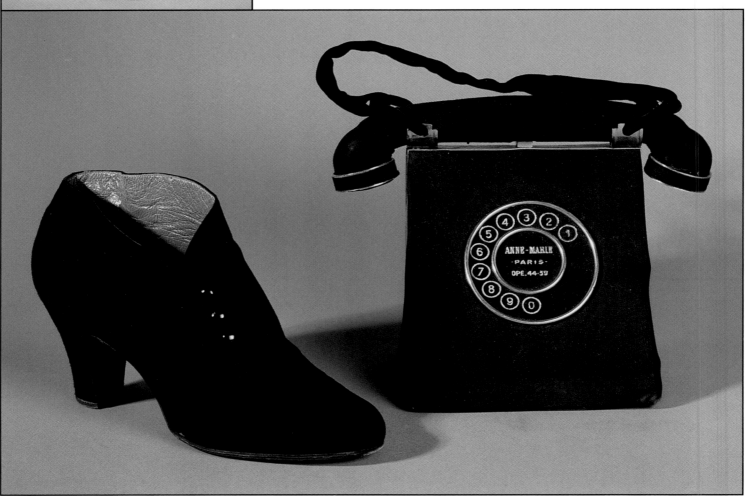

56

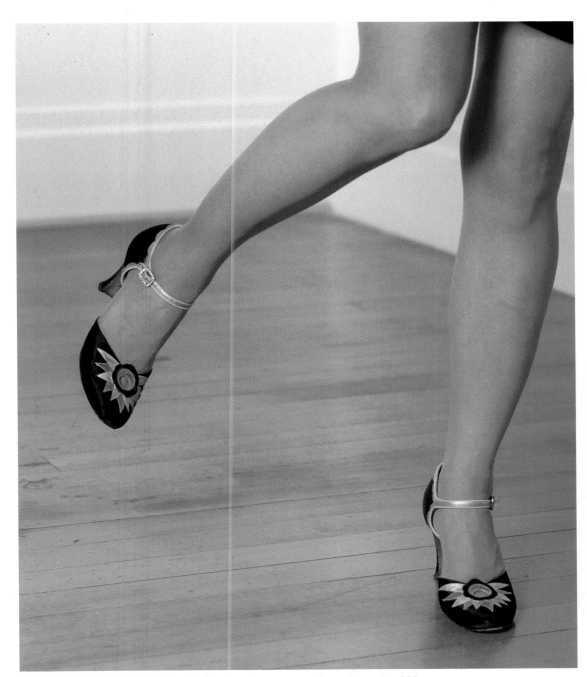

A blaze of gold and silver glorify these dance pumps from the early 1930s, designed by Park-Wolin. *Collection of Sheryl Birkner.* Value: $75-95.

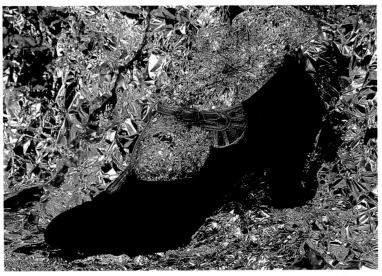

The geometric shapes so emblematic of Art Deco glitter in gold and silver kid on a pair of black sateen T-straps by RoyalCraft, from the mid-1920s. *Collection of Sylvia and Richard Unger.* Value: Special.

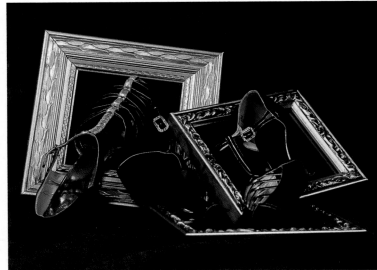

Slinky black satin sandals for dance or dalliance. These shoes stepped out in the early to mid-1930s. *Courtesy of Lindy's Shoppe.* Value: $55-75.

Great Names

EARLY LUMINARIES

André Perugia

The first legendary name in shoe design is that of André Perugia of France. After a brief apprenticeship to his shoemaker father, Perugia opened his first shop at the tender age of sixteen. The year was 1910, when the twentieth century was also young, and ready for a change.

Perugia quickly developed new heels and vamps, some of which would still be considered daring today. At the end of World War I, after Perugia served a military stint as an engineer, he was discovered by the reknowned couturier Paul Poiret. His exclusive, innovative line for Poiret would assure his worldwide reputation.

Perugia would later collaborate with Israel Miller in New York City, with whom he maintained a fifty-year relationship. Perugia also designed for Saks Fifth Avenue, H & M Rayne in London, and Charles Jourdan in Paris.

By the teens, Perugia had a shop on the Rue St. Honoré in Paris. When he opened a shop in New York City in the '20s, it immediately became the premier salon, for society and social climbers alike.

Perugia used only the costliest fabrics, most luxurious skins, and finest leathers. One of his trademarks was hand-painted motifs on leather; another was stamped or pyrographed leather over-dyed for a two-tone effect something like a jacquard fabric.

His was the first celebrity clientele, for whom he fashioned shoes on custom lasts. He designed for Mistinguett and Josephine Baker of the French music halls; for Pola Negri, Gloria Swanson, and Rita Hayworth of Hollywood; and for Queen Elizabeth, along with ladies of her court. In short, Perugia was to shoemaking what Worth was to *haute couture*

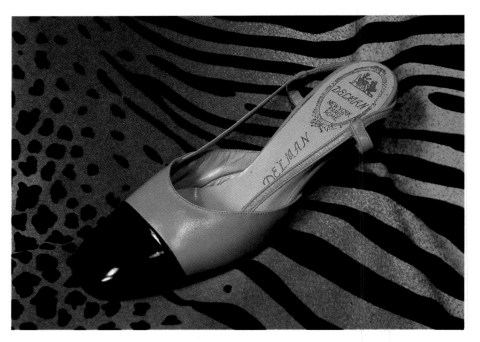

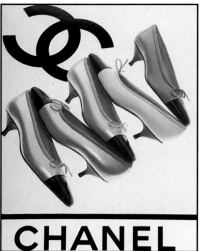

Above: Coco Chanel's toe-cap pump has been re-interpreted many times. She originally designed the style to make her own foot look shorter. Shown, a slingback version by Delman, circa 1970. *Courtesy of Barbara Grigg Vintage Fashion.* Value: $45-65.

Left: Karl Lagerfeld re-invented the classic lines of Chanel for the couture, and boutiques worldwide. In 1997 he postured her patent-toe pump on demi-heels, in sherbet shades of kid. Delicious!

Pietro Yantourni

In the '20s, Perugia's only rival was Pietro Yantourni (a.k.a. Yantourny). An East Indian by birth, Yantourni emigrated to France as a young man. There his interest in the arts and fashion led to a curator's post over a shoe collection at the Cluny Museum. Yantourni only made shoes in his spare time, on a bespoke basis. Only the wealthiest women could afford his wares, at a staggering $1,000 per pair; and only the most discriminating would care to, since he took up to three years to produce a pair. Once he accepted a client, he would cast her feet in plaster, then dispense with further contact until the shoes were delivered.

Yantourni is perhaps best known today by the resonance of his prolonged association with Rita de Acosta Lydig. She was a wealthy socialite of the Edwardian Era, of Latin heritage and New York City birth. Her life was one of studied leisure and a somewhat fanatic devotion to style. He created more than 150 pairs of shoes for her, from her own stockpile of fragile antique laces and textiles, each a small work of art. Lydig's shoes by Yantourni were carefully stored in custom-made leather trunks, and are now on permanent exhibit at the Metropolitan Museum of Art.

Early Labels

Even before Perugia and Yantourni elevated shoemaking to couture status, the world's wealthy and stylish women were beautifully shod. They wore custom-made shoes by Bally of Switzerland and Helstern & Sons of Paris. Both manufacturers had an established clientele by the turn of the century. Both also carried a ready-to-wear line, thus increasing the odds that collectors can still find their shoes at an affordable price.

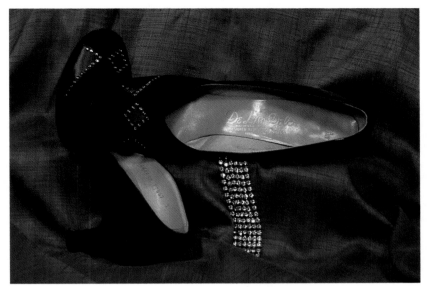

Left: The verve of Palter De Liso is evident in purple velvet and satin pumps. For De Liso Debs, circa 1960. *Collection of Lis Normoyle.* Value: Special.

Below: David Evins designed for the queen, why not for you? His master crafting is evident in these raffia-swirl pumps from the mid-1960s. *Author's collection.* Value: $45-65.

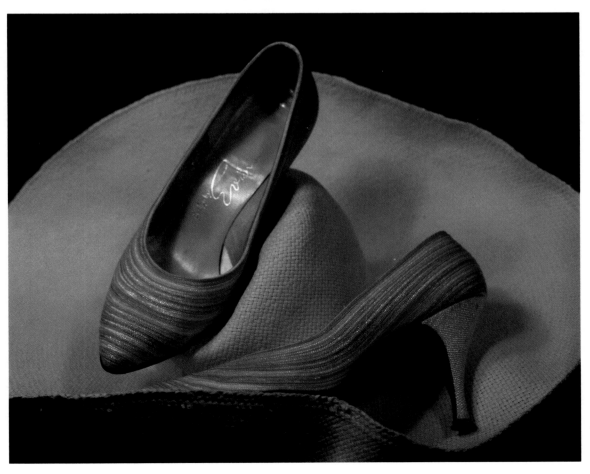

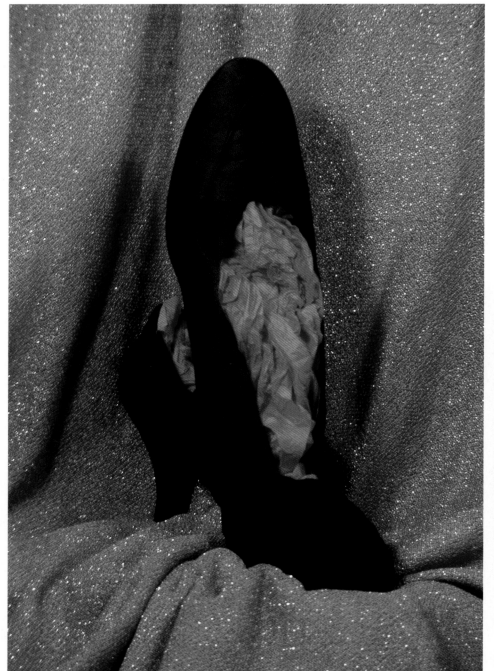

Two jewels in the Ferragamo crown, circa 1975: dress pumps in emerald and sapphire satin. *Courtesy of Barbara Grigg Vintage Fashion.* Value: $35-55 per pair.

SAKS FIFTH AVENUE

1938 Sandal with layered platform sole and heel covered with suede.
Salvatore Ferragamo Museum

Salvatore Ferragamo was one of the most important figures of the "Made in Italy" trademark.
Nicknamed the "shoemaker of dreams", he was the first to export Italian fashion shoes in the 1920's.
From that moment on, his footwear has been sold by Saks Fifth Avenue.
Today, the partnership continues.

The shoe company founded by Salvatore Ferragamo often borrows from its archives of his designs. This advertisement shows his famous rainbow-suede on cork wedge, an innovative design of 1938, next to the stacked heel it inspired in 1997.

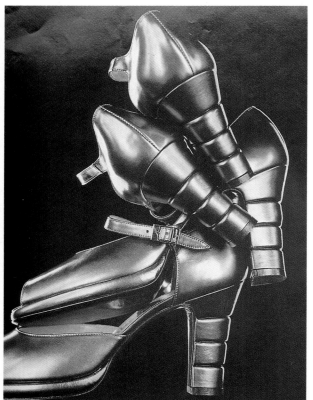

Shoe design took on new dimensions in the '20s, when artisans had access to the advancements of an industrial age. Most of the early design talent was European, but the production innovation was American. There arose a collaboration between companies on this shore (Herman Delman and Israel Miller) and talent from abroad (Salvatore Ferragamo and Roger Vivier). An exception is the Charles Jourdan company of France, one of the first companies that offered luxury shoes to a *pret-a-porter* or ready-to-wear market.

Charles Jourdan, Affordable Luxury

One of the greatest influences on the industry is that of Charles Jourdan, by virtue of his genius for marketing. He was born in France at the height of the industrial revolution, in the year 1883. After overseeing the work of leather cutters in the late teens, Jourdan became an independent manufacturer and introduced *Seducta*, a luxury label, in 1921. Within the next two decades, he created a distribution network throughout France.

Jourdan recognized the importance of licensing and diversification, borrowing these marketing concepts from the great houses of French couture. With his working knowledge of the craft, and his innate business skills, Jourdan envisioned a distribution network that would bring luxury shoes to the broad-based, ready-to-wear market.

After World War II, Jourdan's three sons began running the business. By 1958 they had launched a woman's footwear boutique in Paris, then in London. Ten years later, they opened in New York City.

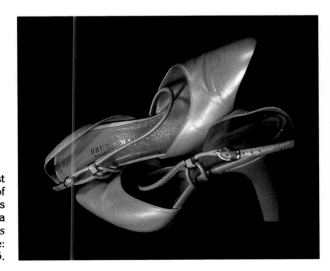

Glacé kid in palest ivory makes a pair of ladylike slingbacks by Bruno Magli, circa 1980. *Author's collection.* Value: $45-65.

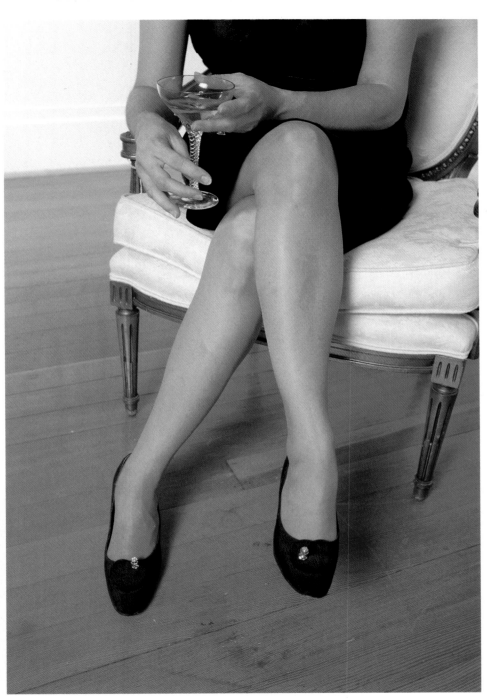

A touch of whimsy from Frank More, circa 1960. His black file pumps sparkle with dew-drop diamonds on a buckle shaped like a fairytale lily pad. *Courtesy of Lindy's Shoppe*. Value: $35-55.

In the late 1950s, Jourdan contracted with the House of Dior for international distribution rights under the Dior label. In the early '60s, Perugia began designing for the company, further ensuring its *cachet*.. When Charles Jourdan died in 1976, his company had twenty-one international franchises, marketing not only shoes but also handbags and clothing.

Ferragamo, Design Innovator

Salvatore Ferragamo is a real rags-to-riches story, in the best manner of Horatio Algier. Born in the early years of this century into a poor peasant family in the Naples region of Italy, he made his first pair of shoes at the age of nine to avoid his sister's embarrassment at the prospect of taking First Communion in wooden sabots!

At the age of 16, he emigrated—not just to America, but Hollywood. By a combination of ambition, talent, and luck he captured the interest of silent film directors DeMille and Griffith. They commissioned Ferragamo to create cowboy boots for Gene Autry, dance pumps for Mary Pickford, and boudoir sandals for Gloria Swanson, and he soon gained recognition as the "Shoemaker to the Stars." He capitalized on this by opening his own salon on Hollywood Boulevard.

Not content to rely on artistic flair alone, Ferragamo went on to study anatomy at the University of Southern California, where he learned that the weight of the body falls on the arch of the foot. With that knowledge, he designed a steel arch support to ensure that his shoes were chic *and* comfortable.

Ferragamo returned to Italy in 1927 and set up shop in Florence, the city of artisans. He created a series of innovative shoe designs over the next few decades and attracted a devoted clientele for both his custom-made and ready-to-wear lines. Ferragamo was also an astute businessman, and was careful to patent his innovative designs (some 350 in all). By the time he died in 1960, Ferragamo had created a fashion dynasty.

The Enduring Legacy of Vivier

Roger Vivier is best known for his collaboration with Christian Dior in the incredible and meteoric rise of that couturier during the decade that began in 1947. Indeed, it almost comes as a surprise to realize that Vivier's was an international career that encompassed many areas of design excellence, both before and after his years with Dior.

Vivier was born in Paris in 1913, and it was there that he studied sculpture at the *l'Ecole des Beaux Arts*. And it was there that he opened

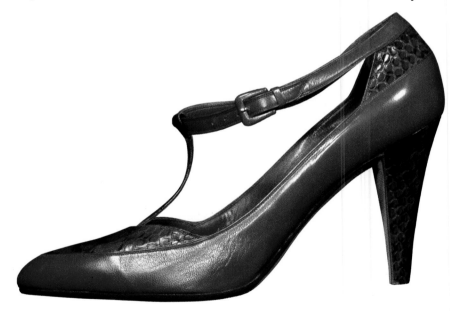

These heels seem fit for a sultan's siren, but they flirted at the feet of a jazz baby. They are stacked spools of hand-turned balsa wood, shod in gold kid. The uppers are black rayon. Imported from "The Beauty Company" in Shanghai, China in the early 1930s. These beauties are now owned by Laurie Gordon, an long-time vintage clothing collector who is active with the Art Deco Society of San Francisco. Value: Special.

The designer Andrea Pfister, something of a shoe sultan in his own right, met Laurie Gordon through a mutual friend in the Art Deco Society. She showed off the spool-heel harem shoes whereupon Pfister begged for permission to buy or borrow them so they could be studied at his atelier in Italy. Laurie reluctantly granted a loan. When the shoes were returned months later, it was with a thank-you gift of red spike heels from Pfister's expensive couture line. *Collection of Laurie Gordon.* Value: Special.

his own atelier in 1937. Vivier immediately began designing for Pinet and Bally in Paris; Rayne and Turner in London; I. Miller and Delman in New York City. (Fortunately for collectors in this country, he designed exclusively for Delman from 1940–41, and again from 1945–47.)

One of Vivier's first sketches for Delman was a thick-soled shoe dubbed the "raft." It was rejected as too avant-garde, but it seems to have suited Elsa Schiaparelli's surrealist sensibilities. After all, she featured raft-soled shoes in her 1938 collection, and is known to have commissioned some of his other designs.

Vivier's career took a brief detour in 1942 when he studied millinery. He went on to operate a boutique in New York City with the milliner Suzanne Remy for the next several years. In 1947, Vivier returned to Paris to work as a free-lance shoe designer. Just in time for the *succès fou* of the New Look!

Of course, Vivier began working for Dior, and when the couturier opened a shoe department in 1953 he was the exclusive designer. (It was the same year as Queen Elizabeth's coronation, for which Vivier designed her modified platform sandal in gold kid, studded with garnets.) During these years, Vivier created a stiletto, and a convex cone or *choc* heel. In 1963, five years after Christian Dior's death, he began free-lancing again and designed for other couturiers like Grès, St. Laurent, Ungaro, and Balmain.

Perhaps because he began his career as an art student, Vivier's design focus was always on the line of a shoe. The embellishment, albeit spectacular, would follow. Using a paper model or *maquette*, he sculpted innovative and aerodynamic heels. Not only the stiletto and *choc*, but also the spool, ball, needle, prism, and pyramid. Perhaps his most legendary design is the *comma* heel. Still in production, it is cast by an engineering firm from the same aluminum alloy used for jet engines.

> "Then there is my darling Roger Vivier, whom I'd known from before the war when he worked here in New York. The shoes he made after he'd gone out on his own in Paris are the most beautiful shoes I've ever known . . . shoes made entirely of layers of tulle, shoes of hummingbird feathers, shoes embroidered with tiny black pearls and coral, all with exquisite heels of lacquer . . . a lesson in perfection."
> —Diana Vreeland, 1984

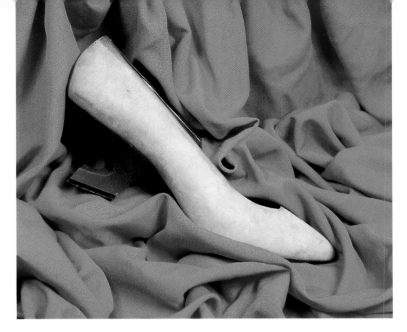

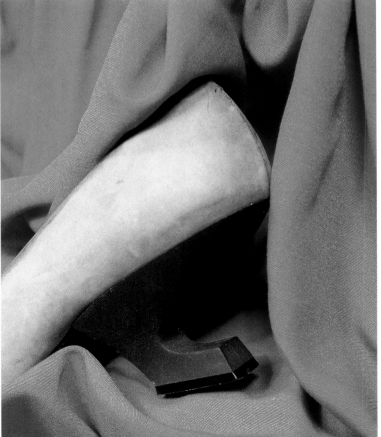

Good luck finding a shoe by Roger Vivier; but knock-offs of his famous styles abound. Case in point: a robust comma heel pump by Sacha of London, circa 1970. *Author's collection.* Value: $15-25.

63

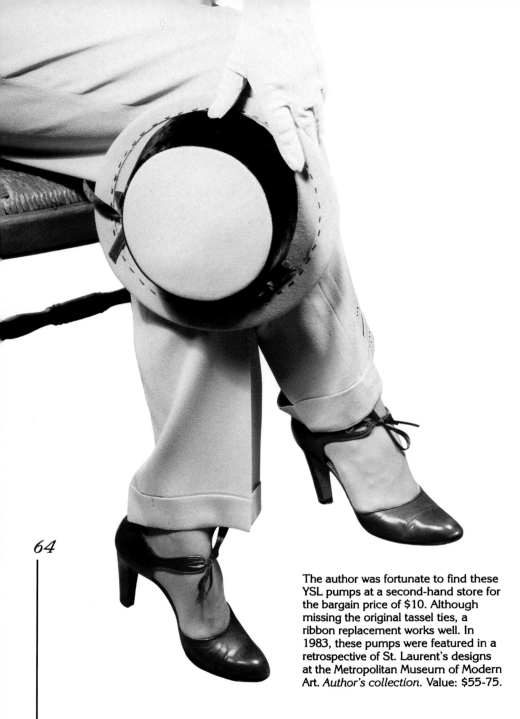

The author was fortunate to find these YSL pumps at a second-hand store for the bargain price of $10. Although missing the original tassel ties, a ribbon replacement works well. In 1983, these pumps were featured in a retrospective of St. Laurent's designs at the Metropolitan Museum of Modern Art. *Author's collection.* Value: $55-75.

David Evins, Quality and Quantity

Ironically, David Evins found his true calling as a shoe designer only after he had been fired from his job as a fashion illustrator at *Vogue* because he employed too much "artistic license" in rendering shoes! He had arrived in this country from his native England at the age of thirteen and studied illustration at the Pratt Institute in Brooklyn.

After the fiasco at *Vogue*, Evins worked briefly as a pattern maker. His talent soon garnered some notable commissions from Hollywood. For example, in 1934 Evins created fantastic jeweled sandals for Claudette Colbert's screen role in *Cleopatra*. His association with Hollywood continued throughout his career, and in 1963 he reprised his role with Colbert when he shod Elizabeth Taylor for the lavish remake of *Cleopatra,* including a pair of gold brocade mules with turned-up vamps that dripped with crystal *passemanterie.*

As with Ferragamo before him, the status of Hollywood was a real boost to Evins' career. He designed sandals for sexy Ava Gardner, one red and the other green, carrying an unmistakable message: maybe yes, and maybe no. At the far end of the romance spectrum, he designed Grace Kelly's pumps for her wedding to Prince Ranier. Other stellar clients included Judy Garland and Marlene Dietrich.

Evins truly launched his forty-year career in shoe design in 1941, with a contract to produce his own label for the prestigious Israel Miller. Just eight years later, he was honored with the fashion industry's Coty Award for design innovation. Evins was the first designer since the 1920s to dye alligator in jewel tones of citrine and turquoise. Even the opera pumps that he designed for Wallace Windsor's tailored wardrobe had a touch of whimsy, like a mix of *faux* leopard skin with black patent leather.

The Evins label was available in custom-order and ready-to-wear in the 1940s and '50s, and he continued designing throughout the 1970s. Given the length and breadth of his career, the label is relatively easy to find (even turning up in thrift stores). For vintage fashion collectors, shoes by David Evins may be the last great bargain!

Labels to Look For

Like the clothes of Dior, so the shoes of Vivier have assumed unparalleled design stature. His *comma* and *choc* heels are almost impossible to find, so eagerly are they sought by collectors and museum curators.

Of course, there are others who employed similar standards of excellence, originality and quality in the design of shoes. These may be the hallmarks of *haute couture*, but as Charles Jourdan proved, they can be found in shoes marketed for a ready-to-wear clientele. We commend the two American designers named below, whose labels are still unrecognized by many collectors:

Palter de Liso created *De Liso Debs, De Liso Couture,* and *Debonaires* . His shoes were marketed nationwide, to the women who frequented Henri Bendel's in New York City, Neimann Marcus in Dallas, Dayton-Hudson in Chicago, and I. Magnin's in San Francisco. De Liso was at the apogee of his talent in the 1940s and '50s.

Every regional market had its own special talent. In San Francisco, it was *Frank More,* whose namesake label was largely marketed through his own store franchise on the West Coast. His most innovative designs date to the 1940s and early '50s.

Certain store labels should also rank high on the collector's list. Consider shoes sold under the "French Room" label for Chandler's; "Fenton Footwear" for Saks Fifth Avenue; "Evins" for I. Miller, and "Mister J" for Joseph Magnin.

Other labels, not overly dear in their day, seem charming and witty today. This category includes Accent, American Girl, Bass, Capezio, Daniel Green, Enna Jettick, Fiancées, Jacqueline, Joyce, Keds and Kedettes, Life Stride, Mademoiselle, Naturalizer, Oomphies, Pandora, Paradise, Penaljo, Queen Quality, Red Cross, Risqué, Spring-O-Lator, and Tweedies.

Unlike their more expensive counterparts, which were sold only in upper-end salons, these shoes peered out from a plate-glass vantage point at the hustle and bustle of everyday life, in every downtown. Picture, in your mind's eye:

- The jaunty bow on a high-heeled pump by Red Cross.
- Red patent for a girl's first heels from Leeds.
- The luster of jeweled mules by Spring-O-Lator.
- Quilted satin, like a housecoat, on slippers by Daniel Green.
- Sneaks in crisp white canvas with the little blue Keds label in back.

These are shoes that have the power to conjure images of mainstream America and that seem to precisely capture the spirit of their times.

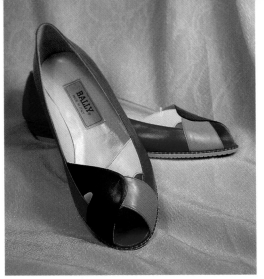

Bally of Switzerland has set a standard of excellence in shoe design and manufacture since 1851, like these glossy multi-color flats from the summer of 1981. It's never too soon to begin collecting designer shoes! *Collection of Harriet Steiner.* Value: Special.

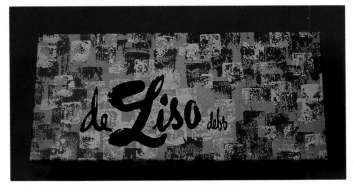

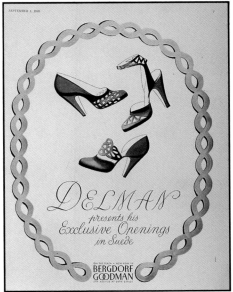

Above: A De Liso Debs shoebox from the 1950s. Also look for the more expensive Palter Debs label.

Left: From Delman in September 1948, Exclusive Openings in Suede.

65

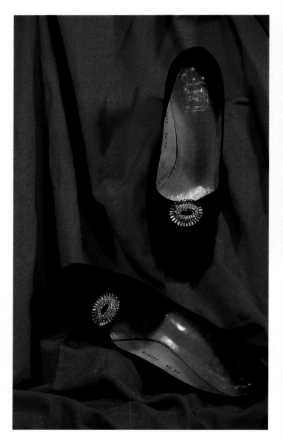

Above:: Black *peau-de-soie* after-five pumps with a baguette clip. Bearing the Dior label, circa 1969. *Courtesy of the Blue Parrot.* Value: $35-55.

Right: Enna Jetticks always marketed "sensible shoes" as seen in this advertisement from March 1955. The company's conservative styles have passed the design test of time.

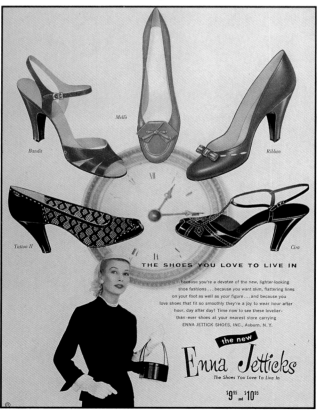

GREAT ASSOCIATIONS

The notion of custom shoes for a couture collection began with Poiret in the '20s when he observed that most of his clients wore shoes by Perugia. But it was Dior's association with Vivier that would spark a real fashion trend. Dior joined forces with Vivier in 1953, promoting made-to-measure shoes under exclusive license. The Dior atelier acknowledged this collaboration with unheard-of name recognition: "Christian Dior Delman S.A.R.L. by Roger Vivier."

Others soon followed in the master's footsteps, notably, his successor Yves St. Laurent, who created designs under the YSL label. In the '60s, André Courreges coordinated his space-age clothes with equally futuristic vinyl shoes and boots, and Betsey Johnson tottered on platforms of her own design.

Today, clothing designers continue to offer a line of footwear in order to assure a perfect complement for their collections. When Karl Lagerfeld of Paris reinvents the classic knit suit by Coco Chanel, he often accessorizes it with a witty take on her two-toned and cap-toed pump. Likewise, the Italian knitwear designer Adrienne Vittadini designs shoes to coordinate with her clothing, sold to an international boutique clientele. In reverse order, shoe designers Joan Helpern and Patrick Cox have added clothing and accessories to their footwear collections!

THE POST—MODERNS

Keep on the lookout for shoes by the best and brightest contemporary designers. They can sometimes be found for a pittance in today's used-clothing market. It's easy to foretell that the same shoes will be sought after by collectors in tomorrow's vintage clothing market!

The names, if not exactly household, should be readily recognizable to anyone who follows fashion trends: Manolo Blahnik, Susan Bennis and Warren Edwards, Patrick Cox, David Evins, Tom Ford, Joan and David, Charles Jourdan, Beth and Herbert Levine, and Andrea Pfister.

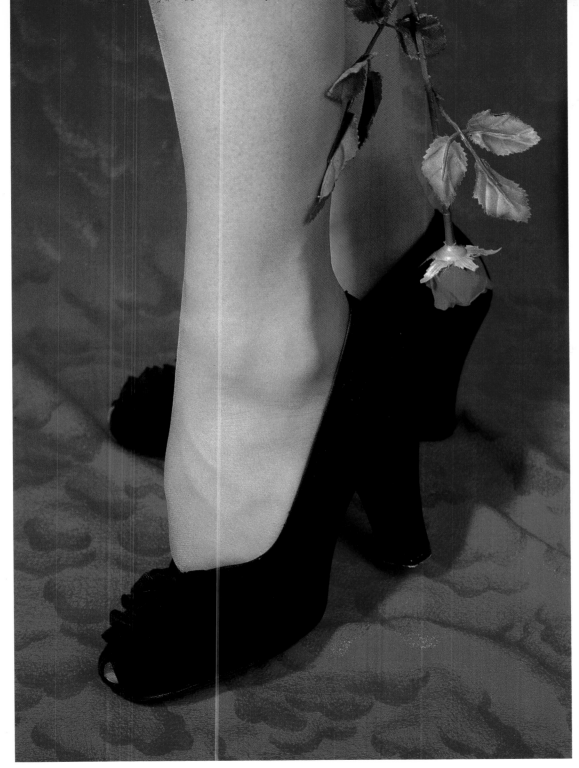

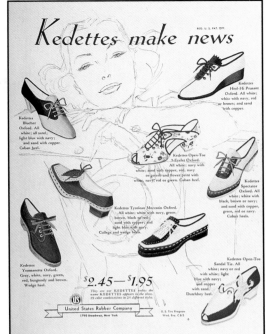

"Kedettes make news." In the 1930s, the company boasted of twenty-nine color combinations in twenty-four styles, priced at $1.95 to $2.45. Kedettes and Keds were manufactured by the U.S. Rubber Company, along with automobile tires!

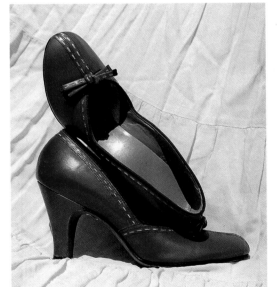

Perfect for a country weekend, circa 1950, caramel pumps with nougat topstiching, new\old stock by Red Cross Shoes. *Courtesy of Lindy's Shoppe.* Value: $35-55.

Left: Fenton Footwear was the exclusive label of Saks Fifth Avenue from the 1930s through the '60s. These peep-toe black suede pumps with grosgrain ruffle are circa 1947. *Courtesy of Lottie Ballou.* Value: $35-55.

Chapter VI

TIPS ON DATING

To properly date vintage shoes, you first need an understanding of the changing role of women in society, as a form of cultural context. Also, the vagaries of fashion and how they influenced shoe design, construction techniques, and the evolution of shoemaking as an industry, offer another clue to dating.

In Cultural Context

Like all aspects of costume, shoe design is strongly influenced by the social mores and political events of the times. For example, a queen's slippers were paper-thin of sole, quite a contrast from the wooden sabots worn by her peasant subjects. It is reputed that the Empress Josephine returned a new pair of satin slippers to her shoemaker, after discovering a small hole, whereupon he explained: "Ah, I see your problem. Madame, you have walked on them."

The changes in cultural ideals that distinguish one decade from the next seem to have caused abrupt shifts in the design of women's clothing. In fact, these transitions were often blurred.

Victorian high-buttoned shoes were correct until the '20s, when they were relegated to footwear for the elderly and infirm. Dress excess in the Belle Epoque was followed by dress reform early in the decade. The first world war brought about an expanded world view, leading to the anything-goes Jazz Age with short skirts and bobbed hair. The second world war brought a series of attitude adjustments. Women entered the work force in tailored suits and sensible shoes. The pendulum swung full circle for a brief fling with Dior's flirty "New Look" before tie-dye jeans and macramé vests ushered in a sort of coming-of-age in the 1960s.

In the late '90s, the tailored look was revived with a vengeance. The look was all about mesh and leather, a sort of biker-chick chic in clothing that was born to be wild with steel-heeled stilettos. Once again, fashion was responding to the social milieu, only this time it was the edginess of a world on the brink of a new millennium.

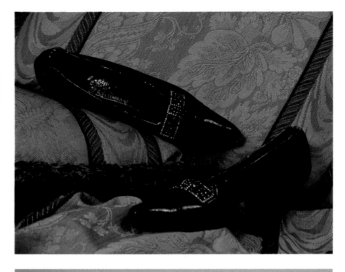

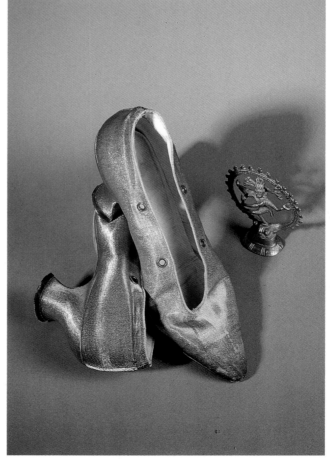

Above: These black kid dress pumps bear the label "Henry Weiss, St. Petersbourg" in gilded script, a telltale clue that they were manufactured before World War I. That was the Belle Epoque, an era of great elegance for the nobility and upper-class in the former capital of Russia. How to reconcile, then, the lack of cording to properly finish the throat of these pumps? Or the marcasite buckle so typical of the 1920s? It is tempting to speculate that these were once dress boots, cut down by an impoverished Russian émigré to stretch her diminished wardrobe. *Courtesy of Banbury Cross Antiques.* Value: $115-125.

Left: Golden ghillies for evening, in the sunset of the British Raj. The fabric uppers are well-preserved, having gained strength as well as glam from a metallic weave. These slippers would have been fastened with ribbons, which may also have held in place a photo of the lady's lover as "an exquisite proof of love and of good taste" according to fashion sensibilities circa 1910. *Collection of Sheryl Birkner.* Value: Special.

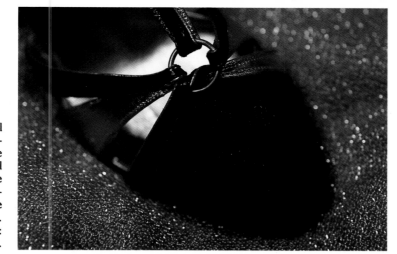

A dance pump in dull black silk with hand-painted gold accents. The gold kid straps and heel add extra glamour. The silhouette and workmanship indicate the late 1920s or early '30s. *Author's collection.* Value: $55-75.

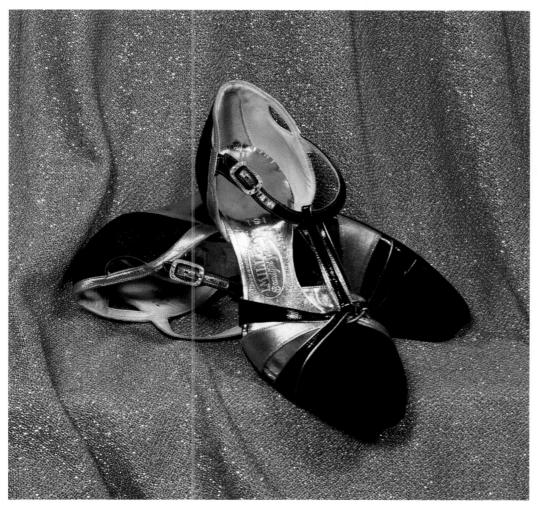

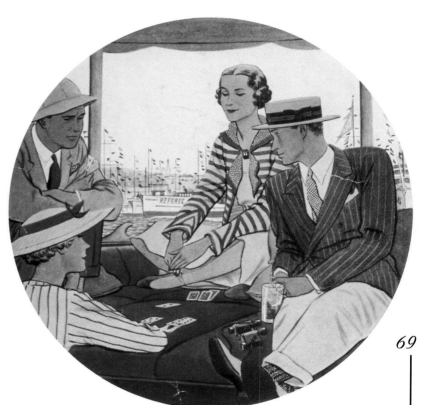

A jaunty young lady enjoys a game of cards, sitting cross-legged and at ease in a nautical outfit and flats. This illustration is from 1934, proving the perennial nature of a flat-heeled skimmer shoe.

69

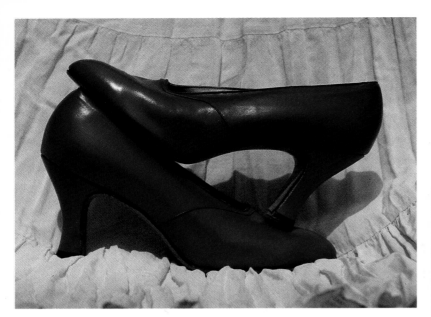

Left: A kiss of lipstick red, just as fresh today as when first worn in the late 1920s. The Spanish heels are a clue to dating, along with the steel arch and leather soles. Inner support for pressure points of the foot are a hallmark of quality vintage shoes, such as these by Feltman & Curme. *Courtesy of Vintage Silhouettes.* Value: $75-95.

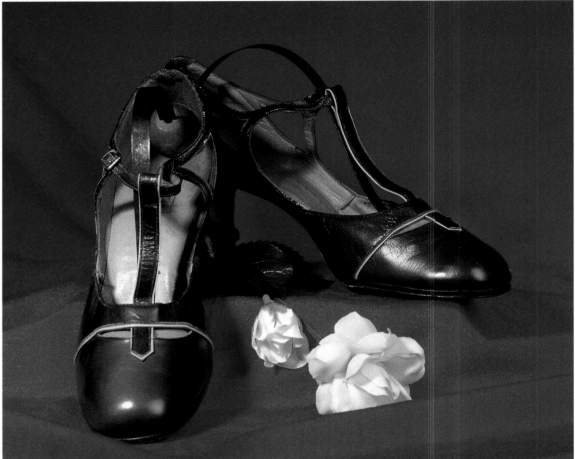

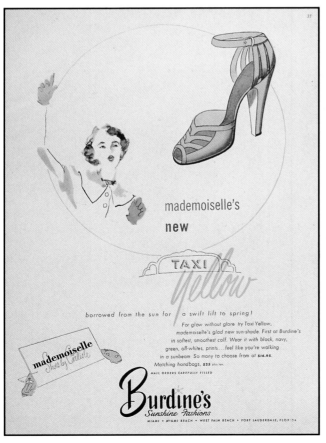

mademoiselle's
new

TAXI
Yellow

borrowed from the sun for a swift lift to spring!

For glow without glare try Taxi Yellow, mademoiselle's glad new sun-shade. First at Burdine's in softest, smoothest calf. Wear it with black, navy, green, off-whites, prints... feel like you're walking in a sunbeam. So many to choose from at $16.95. Matching handbags, $25 plus tax.

mademoiselle Shoes by Carlisle

MAIL ORDERS CAREFULLY FILLED

Burdine's
Sunshine Fashions
MIAMI • MIAMI BEACH • WEST PALM BEACH • FORT LAUDERDALE, FLORIDA

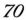
70

Left: When skirts suddenly dropped to mid-calf by edict of Dior's New Look, shoes were boosted *up, up, up* to compensate. Once again, a nicely-turned ankle was a real beauty asset, and it was often emphasized with single or double straps. For Spring 1948, Mademoiselle used taxi-cab yellow to call further attention to city sandals.

Above: What era are they? One glance at the square toe and vivid shade of these kid T-straps, and you may date them from the late 1960s. Take a second look at the fine geometric detailing! These shoes by Wilbars actually date from the late 1920s or early 1930s. *Courtesy of Lottie Ballou.* Value: $55-75.

Clothing Styles

Like all fashion, shoes are subject to the vagaries of taste, good and bad. There is an awesome range between marabou mules and Mary Janes, rhinestone platforms and silver-buckled pilgrims, stiletto pumps and ballerina flats. And yet each style has its disciple, each its devotee.

Consider how the short skirts of flapper fame showed more leg than had ever been seen before, or since until the mini-skirted '60s. This one change in hem lines caused a ripple effect in all other fashions and accessories, as the eye shifted to take in the full scope of new fashions that were adapted to women's changing role.

Be aware, however, that a collective memory of more modest times appears to have lingered into the roaring '20s, demanding the propriety of a closed toe and heel. It was not until the early '30s, that the foot was even partially exposed and then only on certain occasions.

As late as July 1939, the editors of *Vogue* protested: "Open toes and open heels are not for city streets." The magazine admonished its readers that "skeletonized" shoes were only proper for after five, or as resort wear. They were not for city streets, "If you have an understanding of the true essence of smartness, of which the first essential is suitability."

Then there's the matter of proportion, of striking the right balance between a new silhouette in dress with a refined shape to the shoe. For this reason, a new couture collection will often be reflected on the feet of runway models at the Paris and Milan openings. Like the clothes, these quickly filter down to the chain-store brands.

In 1959, two years after his untimely death, Christian Dior's favorite black-and-white hound's-tooth was wrapped around a *choc*-heeled pump by Roger Vivier. A few years later, Vivier styled a simple d'Orsay pump in mod black-and-white mini-checks. The moral of this little tale? If you can't touch an original by Vivier, grab a copycat in tweed or check and you can be confident the shoe was chic in its day.

The changing ethnic influence on clothes can also provide important clues to dating. Think of toe-ring sandals with a nod to Africa; boots trimmed with American Indian fringe; high heels with an overlay of East Indian silver filigree. These were all stock-in-trade for the aesthetics of the new-age '60s. They are to be distinguished from the craze for tropical color combos that marked resort wear in the '30s; a fling with gypsy-inspired pinked and draped fabric, briefly popular in the '40s; or the fad for tooled leather, cowhide, and raffia mixed into a south-of-the-border look that marked play wear in the '50s.

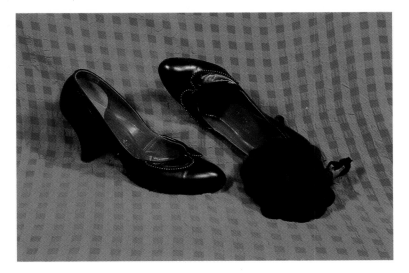

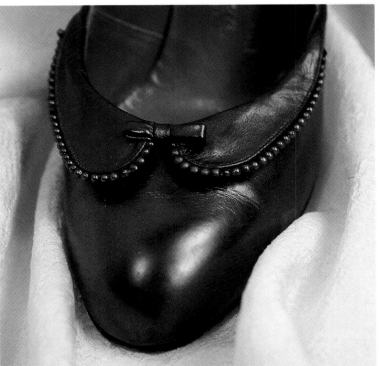

Surely these pearlized plum pumps were worn with a full-skirted lavender shirtwaist, circa 1950, both with a popular Peter Pan collar. The look is enhanced by a sweet bow-tie, and a matching strand of pearls. Sold originally at Saks Fifth Avenue under the store label Fenton Footwear. *Author's collection.* Value: $15-35.

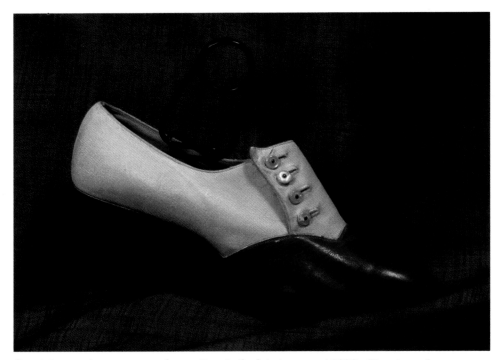

Spectator sports were a popular pastime in the late teens and 1920s. The shoe of choice was a natty tan and white, dubbed the *spectator*. This style is so classic, it is difficult to date. This pump is especially deceiving, since the button closure indicates the turn-of-the-century but the high vamp relates to the 1930s. In fact, it is from the late teens or early 1920s. *Courtesy of Lindy's Shoppe.* Value: $45-75.

The sturdy oxford was named for the type of brogue favored by young men at Oxford University. Its lace-up vamp offers style and support, making it a welcome addition to the active woman's shoe wardrobe as the Belle Epoque drew to a close. The pair shown here dates to the mid-1920s and was hand-crafted in snakeskin by Harran & Son, Inc. *Courtesy of It's About Time.* Value: $65-85.

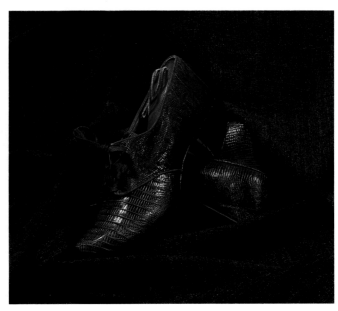

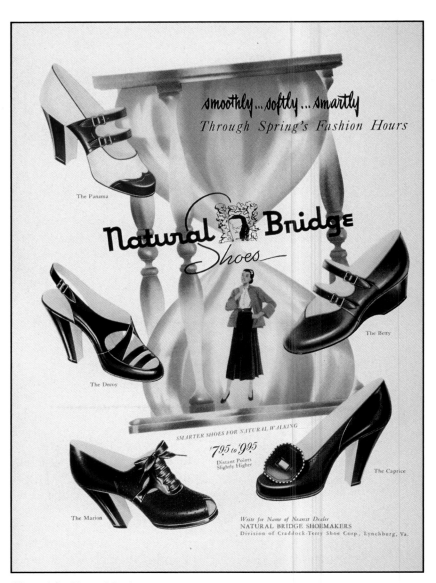

smoothly...softly...smartly
Through Spring's Fashion Hours

The Panama

Natural Bridge
Shoes

The Betty

The Decoy

SMARTER SHOES FOR NATURAL WALKING

$7.95 to $9.95
Distant Points
Slightly Higher

The Caprice

The Marion

Write for Name of Nearest Dealer
NATURAL BRIDGE SHOEMAKERS
Division of Craddock-Terry Shoe Corp., Lynchburg, Va.

This ad for Natural Bridge shoes ran in April 1949, but the high vamps and chunky heels have the look of 1939. It goes to show that shoes are hard to date from the late 1930s to the early 1950s, which is when the leather shortages of World War II began and ended in Europe. There were design "fits and starts" as consumers made do with old styles, from their own closets or manufacturer stockpiles; while designers were creating unusual new styles, from cast-off materials like cork and felt.

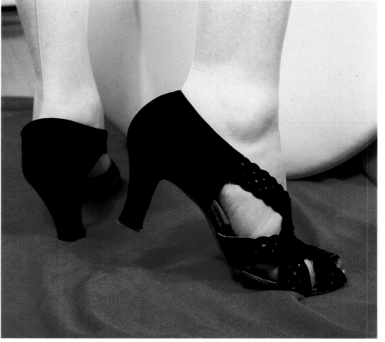

These black suede pumps spelled city chic in 1937, and send the same message when worn by Rhonda Barrett in 1997. This collector seeks out vintage shoes for the special fashion shows that she puts on for local charities, where the models wear clothing similar to Norman Rockwell paintings. The white hatbox in the background is a prop from one such event that featured Rockwell's *Hollywood Starlet*.

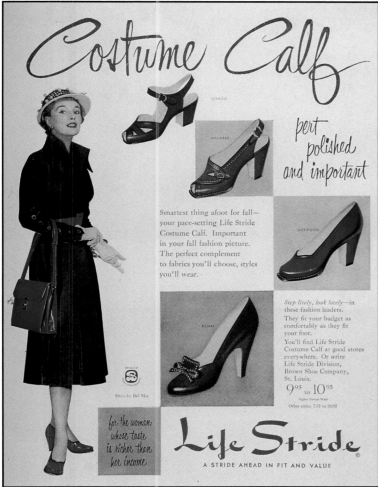

Costume Calf

pert polished and important

Smartest thing afoot for fall—your pace-setting Life Stride Costume Calf. Important in your fall fashion picture. The perfect complement to fabrics you'll choose, styles you'll wear.

Step lively, look lovely—in these fashion leaders. They fit your budget as comfortably as they fit your foot. You'll find Life Stride Costume Calf at good stores everywhere. Or write Life Stride Division, Brown Shoe Company, St. Louis.

9.95 to 10.95
Higher Denver West
Other styles 7.95 to 10.95

for the woman whose taste is richer than her income

Life Stride
A STRIDE AHEAD IN FIT AND VALUE

A slightly slimmer line is seen in these Life Stride shoes advertised in Spring 1952. This mid-price company was less responsive to fashion swings than a couture line like Delman, whose ad for opera pumps that same season was markedly sleek (see page 76). These Life Strides are more suited to a shirtwaist than a chemise.

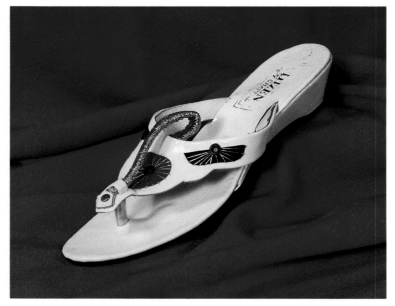

Metallic cording highlights an Egyptian-motif sandal, labeled "Citizen." They may be dated to the early 1960s when the movie *Cleopatra* had just been released. Clothing trends can often be traced to popular entertainment. *Collection of Gail Pocock.* Value: $10-15.

Construction Techniques

For centuries, there was only one way to make shoes, and that was by hand cutting and stitching them. Cobblers formed one of the earliest guilds in the towns of medieval Europe. The Worshipful Cordwainers of London was formed in 1272, its name derived from the town of Cordoba in Spain (which exported most fine leathers). Much like modern trade associations, guilds enforced standards of quality. The Cordwainers are on record as having fined one member forty pence for using inferior leather, in the year 1345!

To be accepted into a guild, a man had to first serve a seven-year apprenticeship. There must have been a long waiting list, because the guild shoemaker was well-off for a member of the working class. When shoemaker John Cams of Cheapside died in 1796, he left 37,000 pounds to charity.

Monied or not, cobblers were among the earliest wave of Europeans to settle in the New World. The founder of the Quaker sect, George Fox, had been apprenticed to a shoemaker. Along with many of his fellows, Fox brought his craft and the custom of apprenticeship with him when he immigrated to Pennsylvania in the early 1600s, seeking to escape religious persecution.

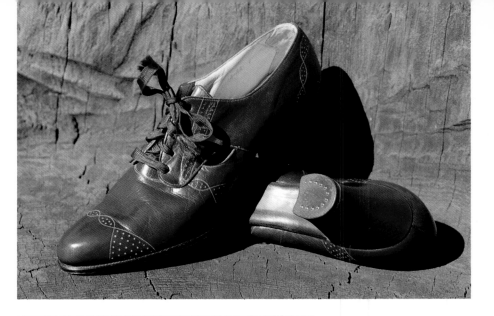

The automatic slide fastener or zipper made its fashion debut in the mid 1920s. It was considered too bulky for a lady's dress, and was used for shoes like these sturdy oxfords from CollegeBred Styles. The zipped oxford remained in style for several years. A similar shoe was featured in the April 1939 issue of *Vogue* : "History will probably record 1939 as America's Walk Year. Sixty miles worth at the New York World's Fair! Thousands and thousands of steps at Frisco! With fashion's rising skirt line more attention is going to be directed toward the foot. You'll relish the scrutiny if you're wearing Grayflex Trampers."

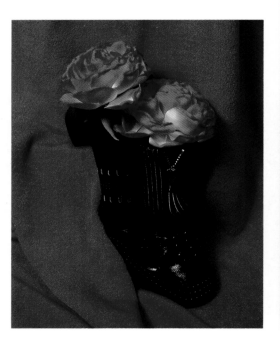

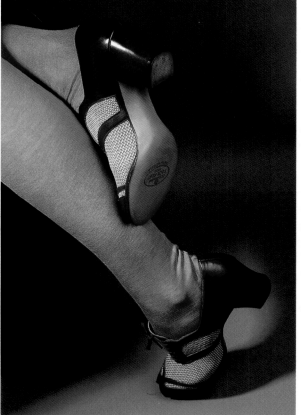

Above: The fine leather and hand-finished soles of these oxfords help date them to the late teens. Note the "finish" of brown leather inserts on the under-sole, surrounding the steel arch. If the heel was waisted, rather than Cuban, they could be dated to the Edwardian Era. *Courtesy of C & L Antiques.* Value: $95-115.

Left: New\old stock is the trade term for shoes that emerge, unsold and unworn, from the inventory of a long-closed salon or department store. The pristine leather sole on these circa 1930 oxfords shows the type of workmanship that is a hallmark of vintage footwear. Note the seamed cotton stockings bagging at the ankle, true to form.

It is likely that Fox knew of St. Crispin, the patron saint of shoemakers. Various versions of Crispin's trials have been passed down by oral tradition. The saint was said to be one of two brothers born to the Queen of Kent in England. When their lives were threatened by an emperor from imperial Rome, the boys were disguised as peasants and sent to Canterbury. There Crispin was apprenticed to a shoemaker and delivered shoes to Ursulus, daughter of the emperor. They fell in love (what else?) and were secretly married. In true epic style, all ended well when the lad's new father-in-law learned of his noble birth and became reconciled to the marriage. The wedding was a secret, but it was openly confirmed on October 25, which remained a traditional shoemaker's holiday.

The earliest shoes were necessarily simple in construction. They were made of a few basic pieces and appear clumsy to the modern eye. But this did not mean the gentry lacked for finery in their footwear. Heels were of leather, pigment-dyed red; uppers were of brocade or embroidered satin; bows were of silk, and buckles of silver.

Surely the demand for luxury will never exceed supply! At the French court of the 1600s, the nobility and hangers-on were known to spend the equivalent of a peasant's annual income on fashionable shoes.

Such fabulous footwear was meant for posturing, not walking. Given the general conditions of mud, muck, and filth that marked roads and streets from 1400–1800, shoes were designed to be worn with leather or metal pattens to protect the sole. The ladies traveled by coach, with little need for their feet to even touch the ground. For short distances, they could go by a sedan chair, and it was considered correct to be carried directly into a room, and so step forth onto a clean floor.

Perhaps the most extravagant court style of the seventeenth century was the silk or satin shoe rose, embroidered with gold and silver and perhaps studded with gems. The poet Roger Bacon wrote: "Now ribbon-roses take such place that garden-roses want their grace."

It was not until the late nineteenth century that common folk could own multiple pairs of shoes, or choose them on the sheer basis of style. Sewing machines and other mechanized tools cut the cost of shoemaking dramatically, though it was still a labor-intensive process. A haberdasher's manual of January 1885 sketched sixteen items that required hand-finishing, for a single high-buttoned shoe. The full listing of pieces was even longer:

"With two soles, two inner soles, two stiffenings, two steel shanks, two rands, a dozen heel lifts, and two sole linings added to the twenty pieces in the upper, the pair of shoes required forty-four separate pieces. Besides this there would be as many as thirty lasting tacks, twelve heel nails, and twenty buttons, making over one hundred distinct pieces, to omit entirely the silk used in stitching the upper and the well-waxed thread which sewed the sole."

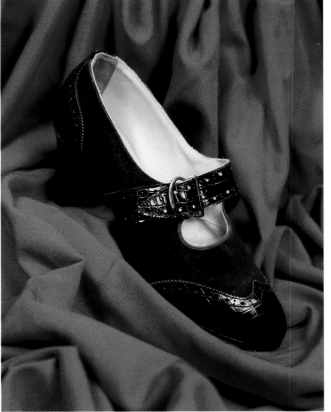

Single-bar spectators in brown suede and leather. When shoes are so classic, they become hard to date. These are circa 1935, as indicated by the steel arch supports, solid brass buckle, and stacked wooden heels. Don't be thrown off by the fact that the alligator is faux, formed by a stamped pattern (see close up). Exotic skins were always pricey and, after all, this was the Depression. *Courtesy of C & L Antiques.* Value: $45-65.

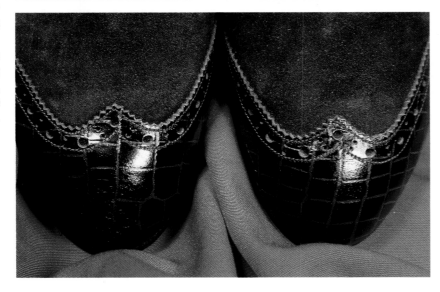

75

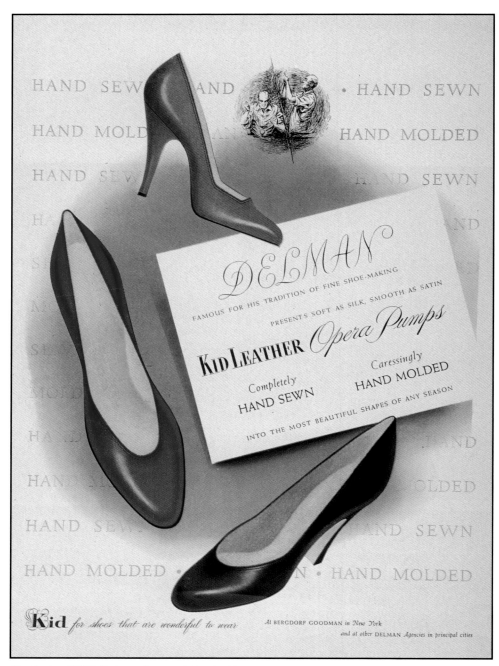

For Spring 1952, Delman featured simple slim opera pumps to complement the New Look. This advertisement boasted "Completely Hand Sewn (and) Caressingly Hand Molded."

In 1892, the Manfield Shoe Company of Northampton, England, perfected machinery to make standard-size shoes in large quantity. In 1858, the American inventor Lyman Blake patented a machine for sewing the soles of shoes. When the Blake machine became commercially available a few years later, a factory worker could turn out three dozen pairs per hour. It was as if the legend of shoemaker elves had come to life, stationed along an Industrial Revolution assembly line.

Mass production greatly affected the shoe wardrobes of the working class, but was barely noticed by the wealthy. They continued to order bespoke shoes, or *one offs.*

In the teens and '20s, and through the mid-twentieth century, made-to-order shoes were also available to a broad clientele. The author's aunt, Regina Glass, is now in her eighties and recalls shopping at a shoe store on Fifth Avenue in New York during the '20s: "I never asked for my own last because the stock fit so well. But it was my regular practice to ask for a leather style to be made up in lizard, or a different color. That was just the way things were done."

In 1950, according to *Vogue*, Evins shoes could be purchased "to order at I. Miller." For an even more custom fit, in 1941 the Henri Bendel department store offered shoes hand-made on their premises, which was just off Fifth Avenue in New York City.

"[W]orkmen and work-benches—without a machine in sight—[it] looks as though it might belong in another land, in another era. But it exists to-day on the premises of Henri Bendel. From heel to toe, the shoes here are entirely made by hand. Made exactly as they were, before the war, by DeBusschére in Belgium. [T]he final triumph of these wonderfully soft, pliable, hand-made shoes—which are ready-made to the American last—is that the price is less than you think."

—Vogue, September 1, 1941

Today, only a few shoemakers have kept the traditional skills of their craft. For a price, bespoke shoes can still be ordered from some ateliers, notably Blahnik, Cox, Pfister, and Ferragamo. There, as in the brief-lived workroom at Bendel's, all steps are performed by hand from carving a last to polishing a finished product—techniques the Cordwainers of London would recognize.

Nothing Is New

Dating shoes of the late twentieth century can be difficult, given a spate of revivals in almost every decade. The most prolific may be dated to the 1960s and '70s, when it seemed that every conceivable clothing style was in vogue for a moment in time.

Like the Jazz Age some four decades before—which also produced a profound change in the way women dressed—the Age of Aquarius was shaped by a post-war financial boom, and a youth-dominant society bent on freedom of personal expression. In both eras there was a resurgence of modernism in the arts and designers began experimenting with new materials and techniques. The 1960s spawned "granny boots" and ankle-strap platforms. The '70s, baroque pumps and pilgrim shoes, with buckled vamps.

How is the collector to discriminate?

Look for fine-grained, glove-quality leather on shoes from the late 1800s through the 1920s. Hand-finished workmanship (such as stamped designs on leather or beadwork on satin) also indicates an earlier shoe. Search for inner construction details like arch supports and brand-name lasts on shoes from the 1920s through the 1950s. Check the label, which is usually stamped into the lining, not just for the name but also to distinguish the thin lettering of an art deco typeface from the bold sprawl of pop art.

Finally, inspect the sole. Is it leather, and does it have a narrow instep with a steel-reinforced arch? Is the heel stacked wood, or perhaps carved Bakelite? Are there thick rubber lifts on the heel tip? These are all signs of vintage shoes. Conversely, a synthetic sole and simulated wooden heel indicate that a shoe is from the '60s, or later.

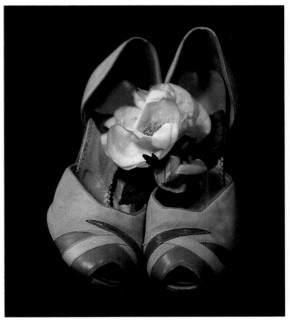

Citrus kid slices are served up on khaki linen platforms with cutaway sides, from the late 1930s or early 1940s. *It's About Time.* Value: $35-55.

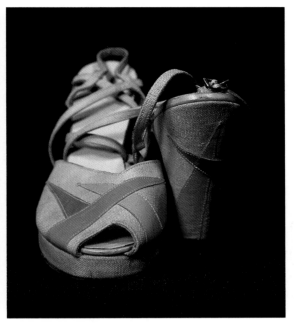

Imitation is the sincerest form of flattery! Similar slashes of lemon, lime, and orange also appeared on suede pumps by Tweedies Alluring Footwear in the late 1940s or early 1950s. *Courtesy of Vintage Silhouettes.* Value: $35-55.

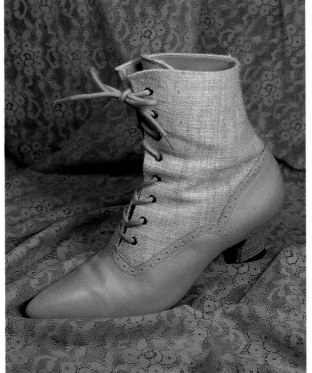

High-button shoes and laced boots from the Victorian era are frequently reproduced by costume companies, and even by regular shoe manufacturers to suit nostalgic clothing revivals. This pair was made by Nine West in the mid-1990s when ankle-length skirts were briefly in vogue. It can be dated as a contemporary shoe by the faux stacked heel (vintage heels were real stacked wood). Also, by the vinyl lining (vintage boots were lined in cotton). *Author's collection.* Value: $15-25.

77

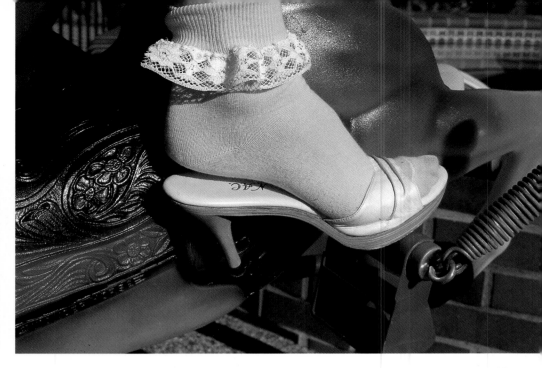

A wooden mule with a single white leather strap. This sexy style was often paired with fishnet hose in the 1950s and 1960s. This style may look uncomfortable, but it came with thick rubber lifts and a cushiony insole. Its contemporary cousin in black faux suede is a throwaway, molded from bare plastic. Bring your own pads! *Courtesy of It's About Time.* Value (left): $25-35.

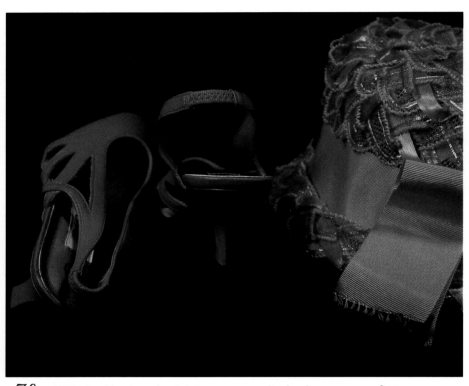

78 With demi-heels and pointy toes, orange slingbacks seem a perfect match for the 1950s straw hat. But these are from the 1990s as seen in the elasticized slings, man-made uppers, and plastic soles. Another dating clue is the label, the house brand of a modern discount department store. *Author's collection.* Value: Special.

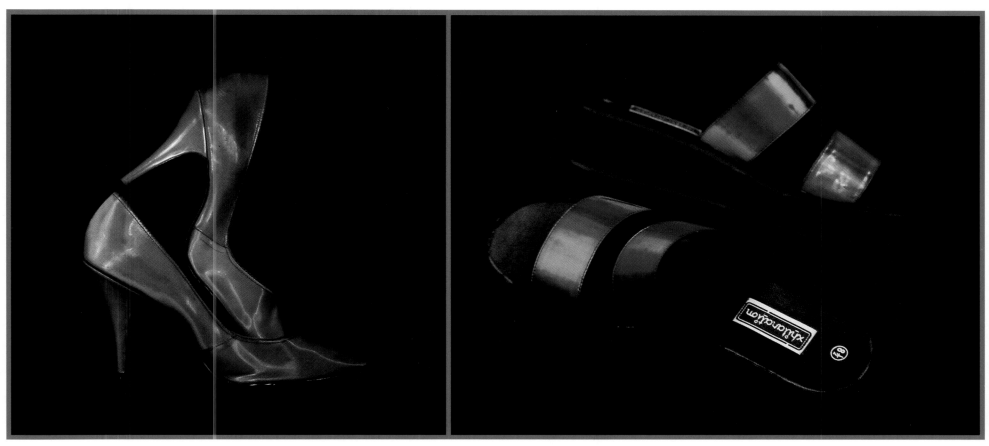

Sunshine and rainbows make a groovy pair of pumps, circa 1965. The same neoprene shimmers in 1997, on sandals that also revive Schiap's raft-soled wedge. *Collection of Gail Pocock, pumps.* Value: Special.

Chapter VII

WELCOME TO COLLECTING

The reasons for collecting shoes are many and diverse. To name a few:

- Fulfill your fantasies in fashionable footwear.
- Enhance your vintage clothing with perfectly-paired shoes.
- Add shoes to your collection of other items by a favorite designer.
- Find a perfect fit in luxurious new\old stock.
- Bask in compliments about your unique personal style.

Enchantments

Women are hard-wired to love red shoes. The lure is so powerful that the moral of over-indulgence, as illustrated in the ballet *The Red Shoes*, is really no deterrent at all.

Then too, the fairytale charm of a glass slipper. Did the fairy godmother have vinyl cocktail mules in mind, when she shod the girl in glass? Perhaps not, but it's safe to say that every woman has a Cinderella moment when she slips into an invisible shoe.

For real shoe lovers, there's nothing like a good boot. Made for walking, or just for basking in compliments, short and sassy or thigh-high, out of leather, cloth, or vinyl, closed by zipper, buckle, or laces—style it any way at all, the boot is a shoe-in.

FANTASY IN RED

One of the author's earliest memories was destined to form a life-long passion for shoes in the shade and glaze of a candied apple. It involved a tearful episode at the Red Goose store, where her mother insisted on buying sturdy brown oxfords for the first day of Kindergarten, instead of red patent Mary Janes with black ribbon bows.

Even the gift of a candy-filled goose egg did nothing to ease the pain. How many women among the readers of this book could tell a similar story? Who among us is still searching for the lost dreams of childhood in the gloss of red patent shoes?

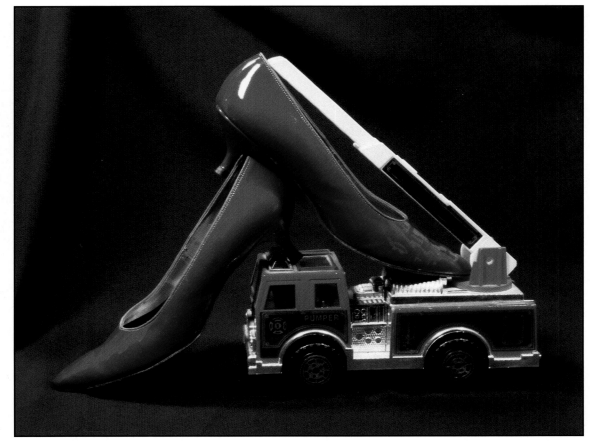

Fire-engine red vinylized kid forms a low-slung silhouette like Audrey Hepburn wore in *Funny Face* in 1957. These pumps are by Rhythm Step. *Courtesy of It's About Time.* Value: $15-25.

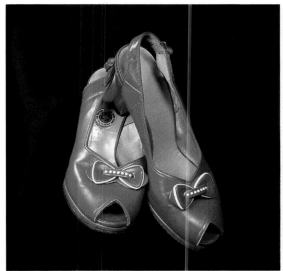

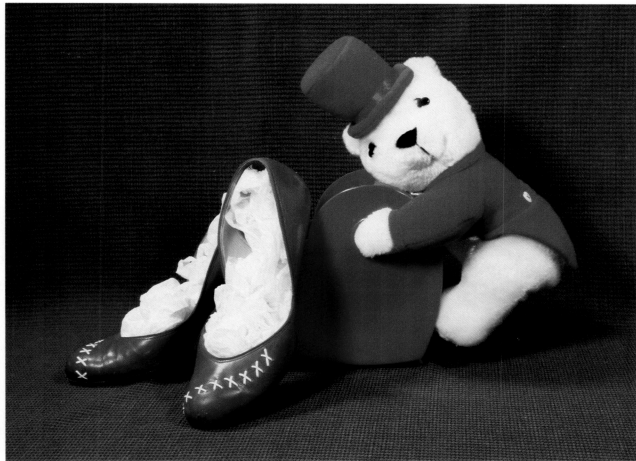

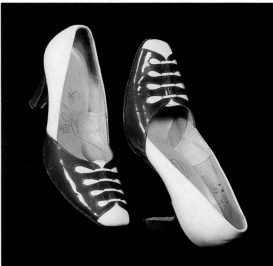

Above left: Red kid slingback pumps by Red Cross, circa 1940. The spiffy bowties are piped in white kid, then pinned in place with a pearl bar. *Courtesy of Cheap Thrills.* Value: $25-45.

Above right: White "kisses" run around the vamp of a Valentine shoe from the early 1950s. *Courtesy of Lottie Ballou.* Value: $15-25.

Left: Mock braiding parades up the vamp of these vinylized kid pumps—a smart stepper from the early 1980s by Johansen. *Courtesy of Cheap Thrills.* Value: $15-25.

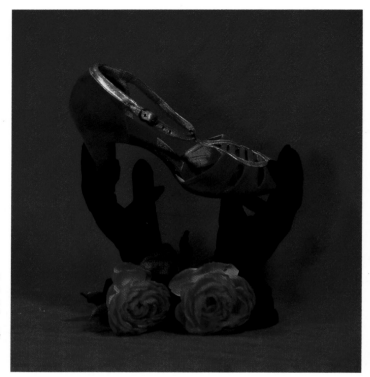

Jazzy red velveteen dance sandals are strapped in place with gold kid; by QualiCraft, circa 1935. *Courtesy of Lindy's Shoppe.* Value: $55-75.

Stark chic in red and black, note the bead edging around the black kid "coins" on this spike-heel pump by Jocelli. *Courtesy of It's About Time.* Value: $15-25.

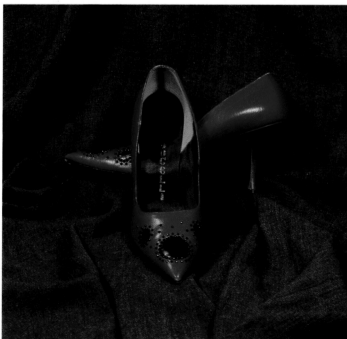

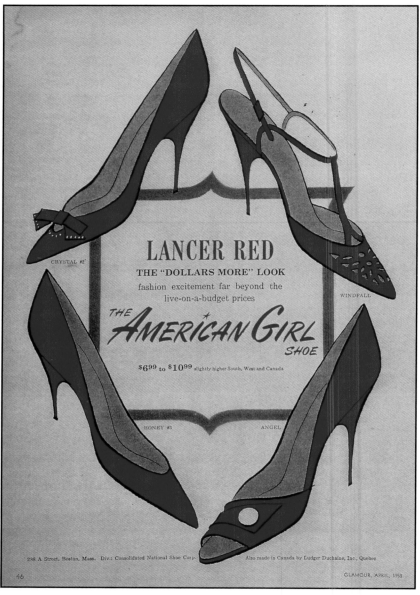

LANCER RED
THE "DOLLARS MORE" LOOK
fashion excitement far beyond the live-on-a-budget prices

THE *American Girl* SHOE

$6⁹⁹ to $10⁹⁹ slightly higher South, West and Canada

CRYSTAL #2

WINDFALL

HONEY #3

ANGEL

288 A Street, Boston, Mass. Div.: Consolidated National Shoe Corp. Also made in Canada by Ludger Duchaine, Inc., Quebec

46

GLAMOUR, APRIL, 1958

A quartet of lissome Lancer Red high heels were advertised by *The American Girl* for spring 1958.

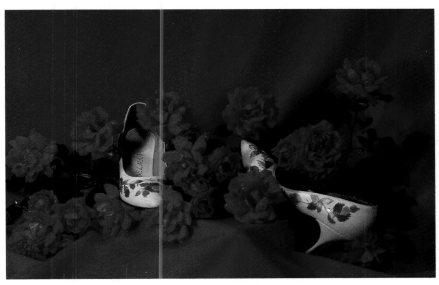

Brilliant red raffia roses bloom in gay profusion on white kid spike-heel pumps by Delman, so realistic you can almost smell the summer breeze of 1960. *Courtesy of Luxe.* Value: $15-25.

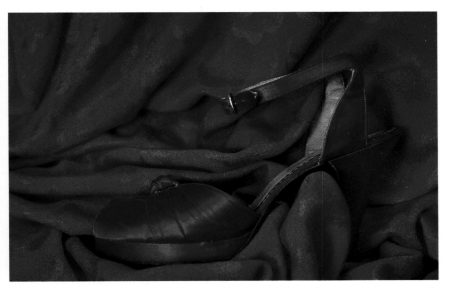

Siren shoes in flaming satin by Stylepride from the mid 1940s. *Collection of Connie Beers.* Value: Special.

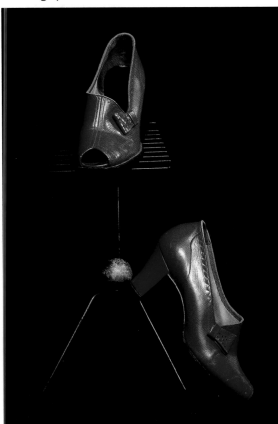

Sporty pumps with mock side buckle, perfect for walking about town and country, circa 1930. *Courtesy of Vintage Silhouettes.* Value: $35-55.

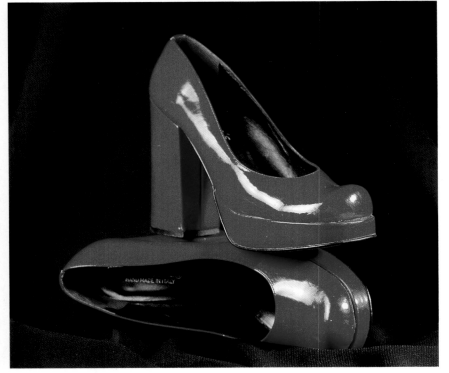

Really red revival platforms! These big, bold, and beautiful patent pumps were made in Italy, circa 1975, by Famolare for the Bibiana's label. *Courtesy of Lindy's Shoppe.* Value: $150-175.

CINDERELLA STORY

When leather was reserved for soldier boots in World War II, shoemakers made do with a variety of substitutes like wood, cork, felt, straw, and fabric. From this necessity of wartime, many new styles emerged. Perhaps the most enduring is the synthetic vinyl slipper, like a fairytale from the pages of fashion history.

It is most commonly attributed to Ferragamo. As the story goes, he was inspired by watching fishermen casting nets into a river, shortly after the war. From this idyll, he created the invisible shoe in 1947, when the war was over but materials were still scarce in Europe. Ferragamo literally took strands of nylon fishing line, and fastened them to a wooden wedge-sole covered in red calf.

Vivier designed in vinyl shortly after the war, for Delman. It was a look he would revive in the '60s, creating an entire collection in vinyl for his own designer label. The glass slipper is also associated with Beth and Herbert Levine for their clear, low-heel pump lined in silver, a perfect complement to vinyl minis in the mid-1960s.

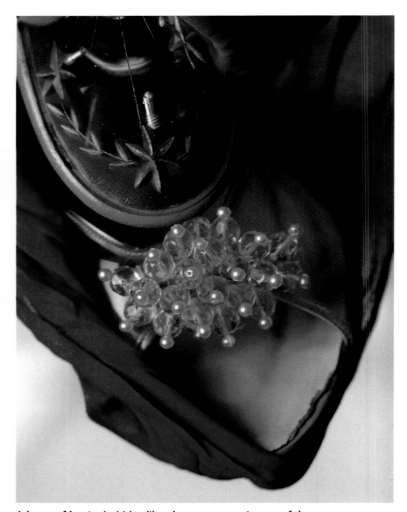

It's in the bag, vinyl and Lucite shoes from the 1950s glowing with silver kid and rhinestones. The style was so popular in its day, collectors should have no problem finding them in good repair. *Courtesy of Lottie Ballou.* Value, each pair: $15-35.

A burst of Lucite bubbles like champagne at the toe of these see-through sandals, made even more festive with a carved Lucite heel, circa 1955. *Author's collection.* Value: $25-35.

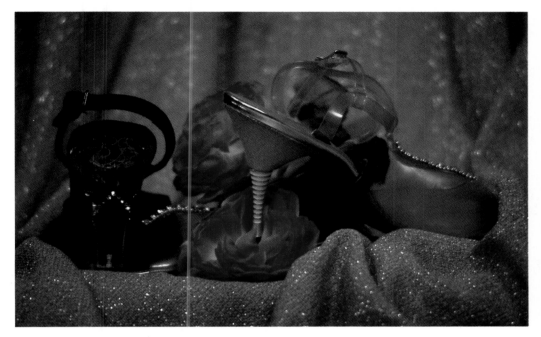

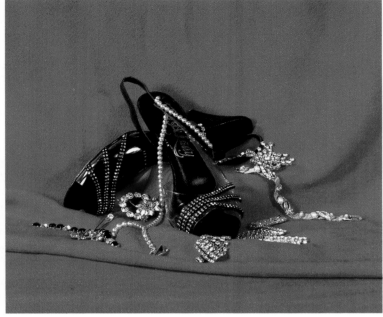

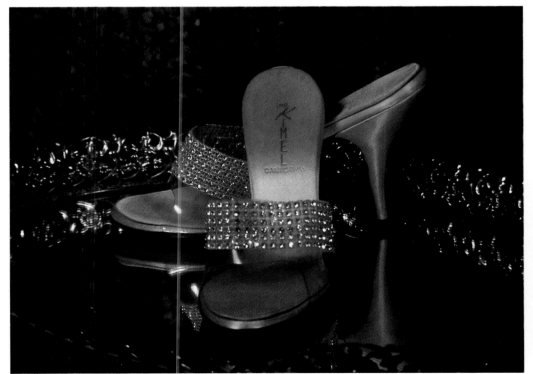

Above left: The heels have it in carved and metal-banded Lucite, for the cocktail party circuit circa 1955. *Courtesy of It's About Time.* Value: $15-35.

Above right: Rhinestones are forever on the Lucite heels of clear vinyl and black silk twill sandals. By L.A. Lady, circa 1955. *Collection of Gail Pocock.* Value: $15-25.

Left: Who wouldn't preen in the looking glass when wearing glass slippers such as these? Satin-heeled mules are pristine if not pure in old\new stock. By Mr. Kimel, circa 1955. *Courtesy of Vintage Silhouettes.* Value: $25-35.

85

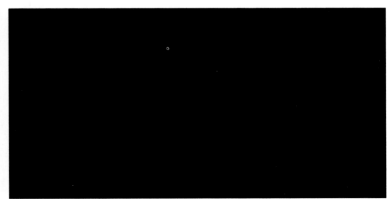

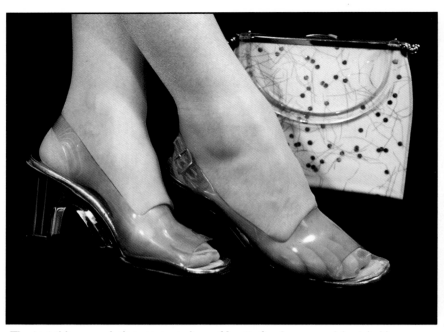

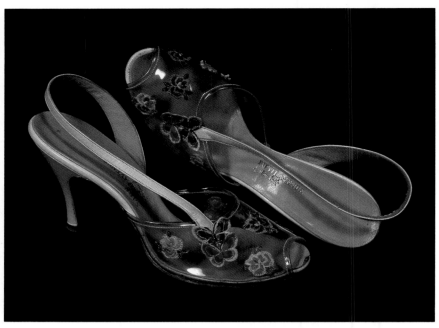

The invisible vamp balances on a sliver of Lucite for dressy sandals styled by Jack Rogers in the mid-1950s. *Collection of Rhonda Barrett.* Value: Special.

Butterflies fly freely on a clear vinyl vamp. Slingback sandals circa 1959, by Fenton Footwear for Saks Fifth Avenue. *Courtesy of It's About Time.* Value: $25-55.

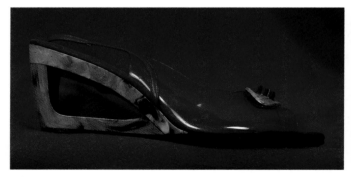

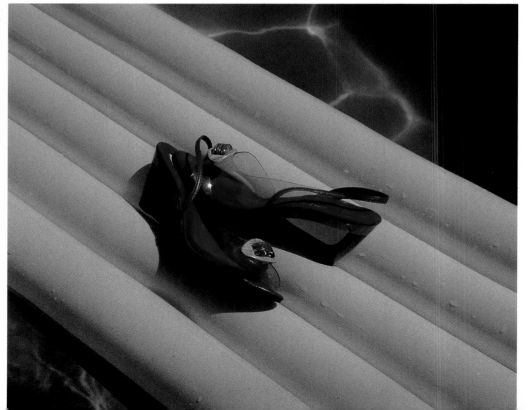

Above & Right: The pierced wedge designed by Perugia in the early 1940s has been copied many times over for mass consumption. This playful pair is by Dezario, with a molded plastic wedge and mock buckle. They can be dated as a revival style from the 1960s, given the use of plastic rather than Lucite or Bakelite. Value: $15-25. Author's collection.

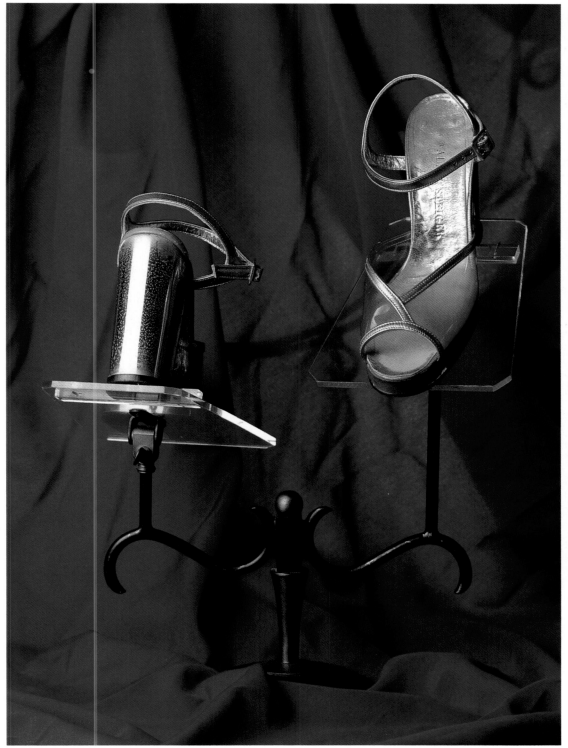

Gold kid wraps up a sliced orange vamp, and serves it on the chunkiest of heels. Wild platforms for disco-dancing in the 1970s. *Courtesy of Lindy's Shoppe*. Value: $110-125.

GETTING THE BOOT

Boots may be meant for walking, but they became fashion standouts along the way. Like no other form of footwear, boots provide a vast expanse of surface area for embellishment and easily set the theme for an ensemble.

Boots swagger and dash, leap and prance, and reek of romance and adventure. Chopped to the ankle, fringed and pinked, they were a touch of fantasy for Perugia. Trimmed with fur by Yves St. Laurent, they were the underpinning of his Cossack collection. Stretched out thigh-high in silvered vinyl by Roger Vivier, they strode into the Sexy Sixties.

Originally, boots were strictly masculine, the gear of soldiers and pirates and other dashing fellows. The thigh-high *cuissarde* is perhaps the most adventuresome, worn by musketeers and soldiers-of-fortune. In fact, the term "booty" comes from their usage by smugglers, who stashed contraband in them!

Women first began wearing boots in the mid-1800s, in a low-heeled style that laced up the side and stopped at the ankle. Queen Victoria kept the look alive when she sported about her beloved highlands in a higher, front-laced boot of cream and tan leather. (This style is still known as the Balmoral, after her castle in Scotland.) Later in her reign, the Victorian woman would wear high-button shoes with the look of a boot to ensure modest coverage of leg and ankle. Ironically, this corset-like closure created one of the most coquettish styles of footwear ever known.

Flower power boots lace-up in lavender suede, with machine embroidery at the sides. *Courtesy of Luxe.* Value: $65-95.

88

These butter-yellow suede boots feature cut work, suitable for the ethnic fashions of 1965. But don't walk in the rain or snow! *Courtesy of Cheap Thrills.* Value: $45-65.

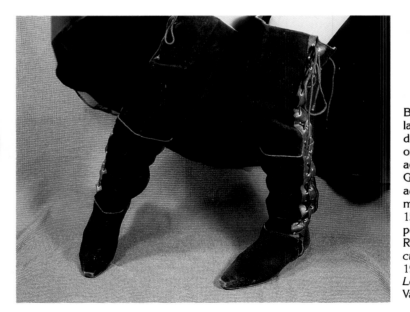

Black suede boots lace up the thigh, derived from a style originally worn by actors in ancient Greece. They were adapted by musketeers in the 1560s, and popularized by Roger Vivier as *cuissardes* in the 1960s. *Courtesy of Lottie Ballou.* Value: $75-95.

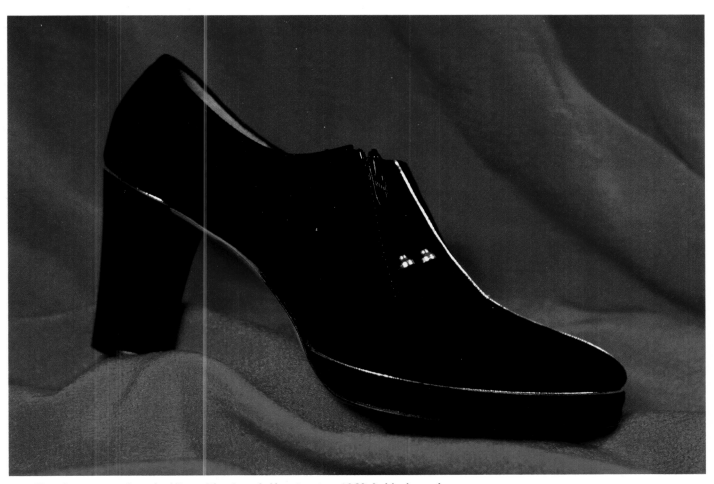

The classic pants boot by Mister J for Joseph Magnin, circa 1960. In black suede with gold kid cording and tassel detail. *Courtesy of Cheap Thrills.* Value: $45-65.

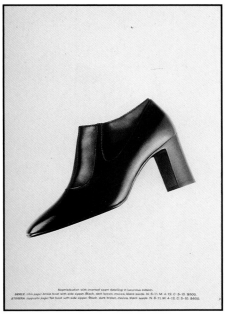

In 1997, Bally featured a very similar pants boot in black kid.

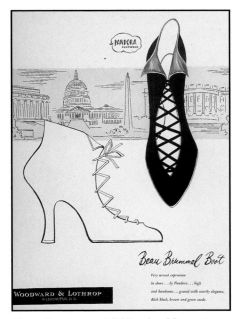

From Pandora in 1950, adorable pants boots laced with medieval magic.

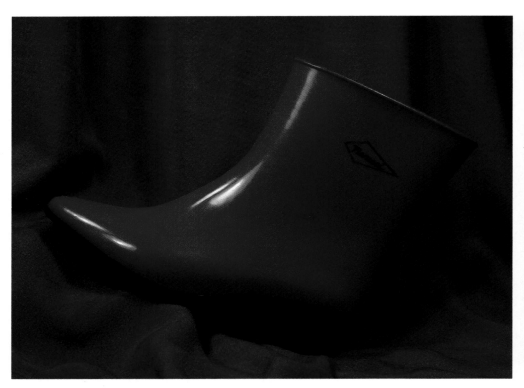

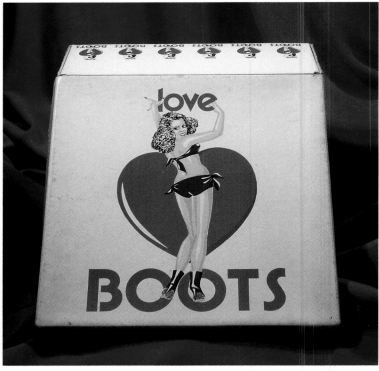

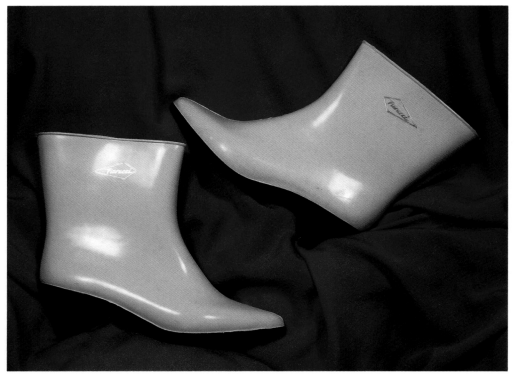

Playful and youthful, molded rubber rain boots from the Italian firm Fiorucci in two colors, along with the original box, circa 1965. *Author's collection.* Value: $15-35.

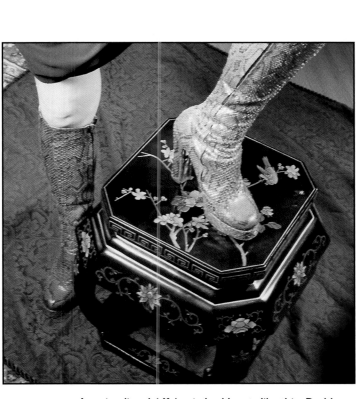

Leaping lizards! If Annie had boots like this, Daddy Warbucks would have been more attentive. A pair of python platforms strutting on four-inch heels, circa 1969. *Collection of Lis Normoyle.* Value: Special.

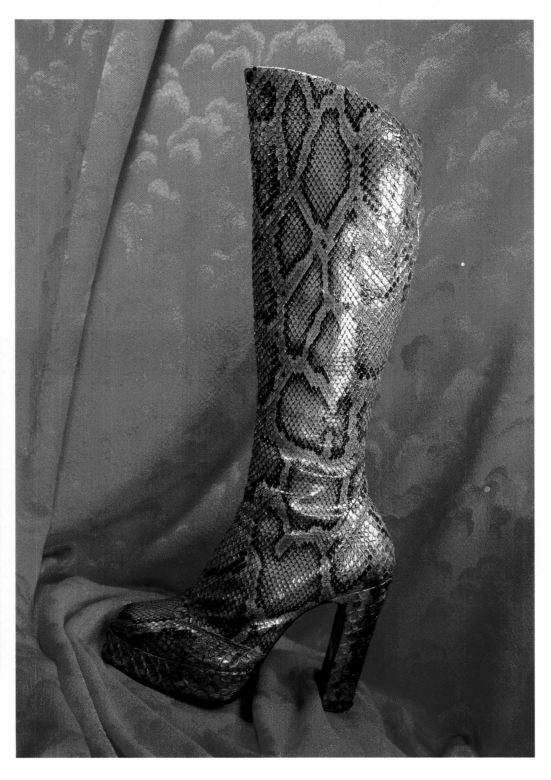

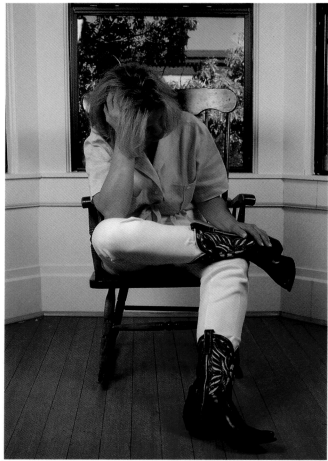

Genell Durkee ponders the next purchase for her show-based vintage fashion business, in a pair of dude-ranch boots. "I don't really specialize in shoes, but I'll snatch them up if they're great, especially new\old stock." Not that you'd know it from her relaxed pose in this photo, but Genell admits to great excitement when the right shoes walk across her path.

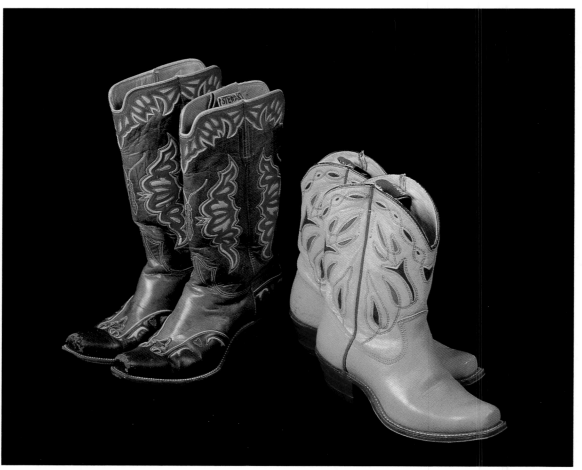

Western boots are a specialized collectible. The finest vintage examples are lavishly designed and custom-made in a mix of exotic leathers. They sell for record prices at auction. The hand-finished variety, circa 1955, such as the cowgirl boots shown, are still affordable in the $150-200 price range. The turquoise pair are from Stewart Romero, the yellow pair are attributed to the Hopalong Cassidy label. *Courtesy of Pamela Joyce.*

Enhancements

The treasures of Ali Baba may lay at your feet in the form of beaded, jeweled, and gilded shoes. They are a perennial bloom in the evening wear garden. The cost of hand-beading makes this the rarest of the species, but jeweled shoes are as plentiful, and sweet underfoot, as wild mint. (In the '20s, *diamonté;* in the '50s, rhinestones; in the '70s, one bold acrylic.) Gilding in gold or silver has graced evening shoes since the 1880s and is used now to spark daytime looks.

BEADED

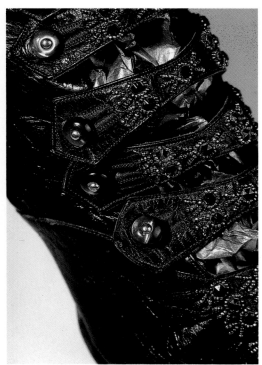

A multiple barrette boot from the Belle Epoque, resplendent with gold beads sewn by hand. This type of boot would have been worn to dinner or theater, with an equally splendid beaded and bustled gown. From the firm of Carnmeyer in New York City. *Collection of Viola de Cou.* Value: Special.

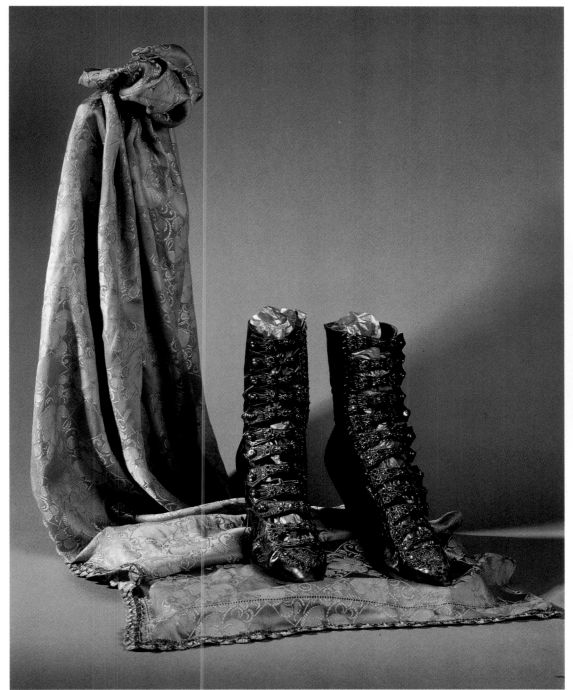

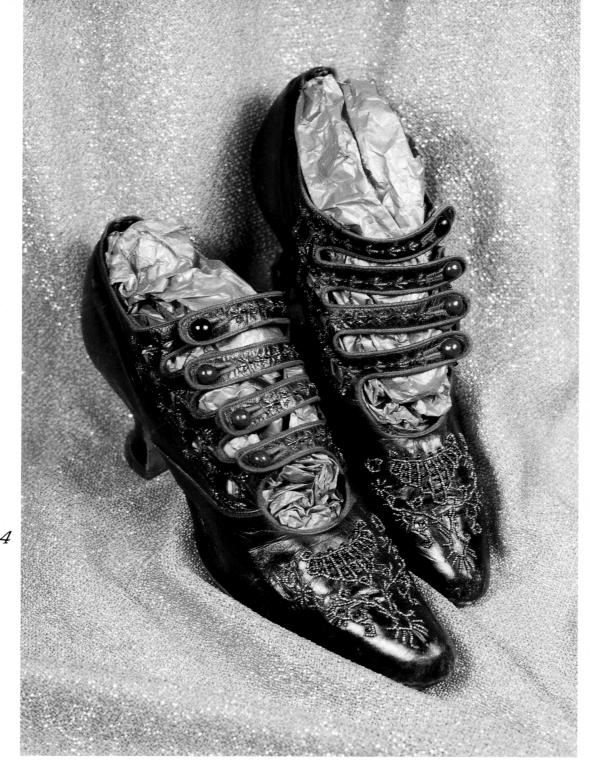

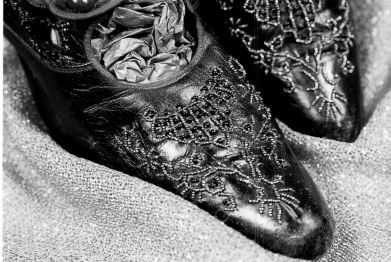

These multi-bar shoes are in crushable glove kid in a shade of eggplant that was fashionable around 1915. The painted wood brown buttons are original to the shoe, in the same hue as the buttonhole twist. The waisted heel is relatively high, a trend that would continue into the 1920s. *Courtesy of Luxe.* Value: $125-135.

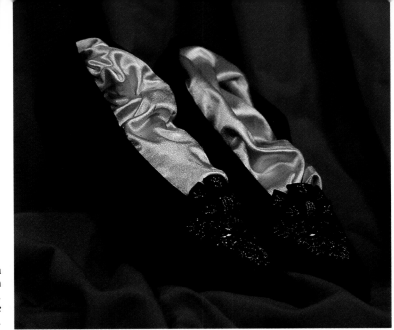

These court shoes feature a ribbon cockade and lavish jet beading, circa 1918. *Courtesy of The Blue Parrot.* Value: $135-155.

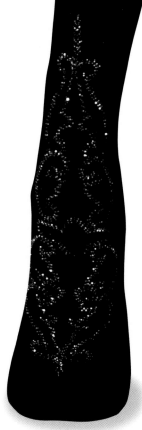

The rise of hem lines in the teens and twenties made ankles into an erogenous zone! Fancy stockings, such as these in beaded black silk, were used to good advantage by ladies with a delicately-turned ankle. *Collection of Carol Sidlow.* Value: Special.

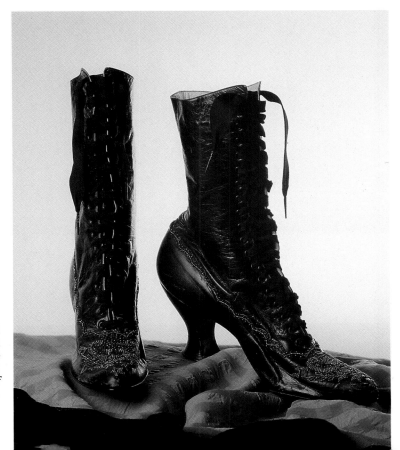

From the Gay Nineties, high-laced black kid boots glitter with marcasite beading. Custom-made for the carriage trade by J. & T. Cousins, New York. *Collection of Carol Sidlow.* Value: Special.

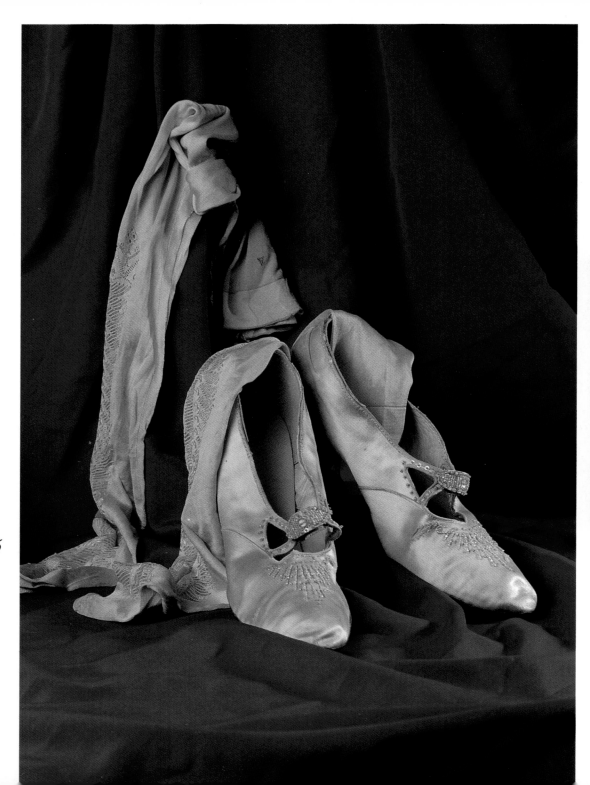

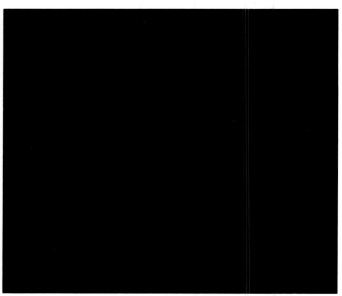

These ivory satin single-bar shoes have a low-waisted Louis heel (not shown), from the late teens. They feature white glass beading sparked with a cabochon rhinestone, and would have been worn with fancy silk stockings like the pair shown. *Shoes courtesy of Lottie Ballou, Bernicia, CA; stockings of Carol Sidlow.* Value: shoes, $115-135; stockings, special.

White satin dance pumps with clear glass beads and rhinestones forming a stylized floral motif on the vamp. The emerging influence of art deco is clear in this design from the early 1920s by The Koenig Shoe Co. of San Francisco. *Author's collection.* Value: $95-115.

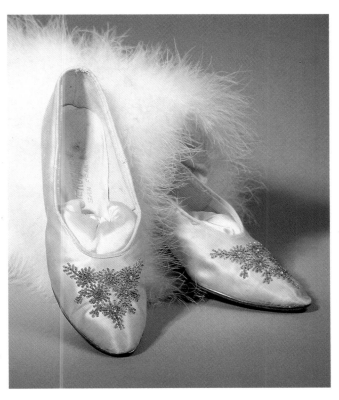

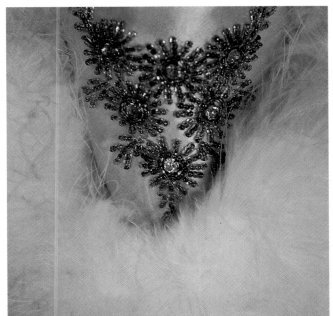

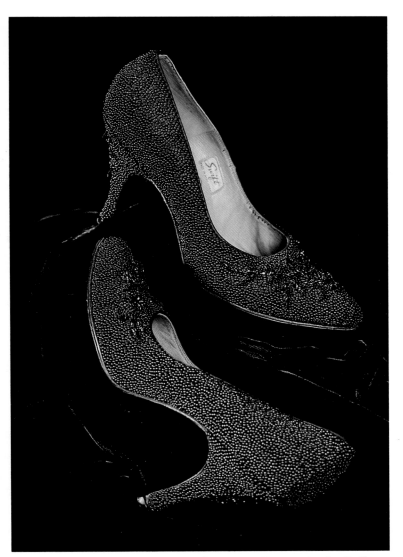

This late 1950s pump was imported from Hong Kong under the Swift label. It shows the kind of hand workmanship that was already prohibitively expensive in this country. The allover glass beading creates black magic for a gala evening. *Courtesy of Lottie Ballou.* Value: $75-95.

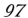

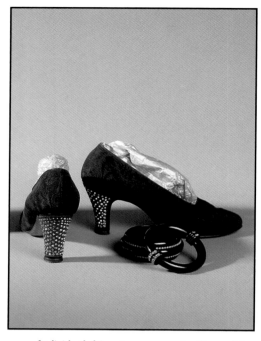
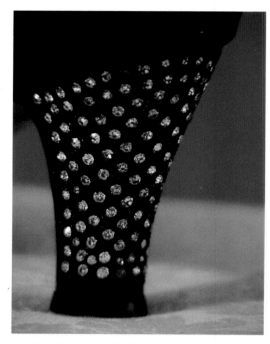

Individual rhinestones are set with precision in the Bakelite heels of silk brocade opera pumps by Sommer & Kaufman, from the late 1930s or early 1940s. This technique was also popular in jewelry from the same era. *Courtesy of Lottie Ballou.* Value: $95-115.

JEWELED

In 1988, MGM auctioned the ruby slippers worn by Judy Garland in *The Wizard of Oz.* The winning bid was a red-hot $187,000. A small price to pay, though, considering that the legendary jeweler Harry Winston later made a commemorative jeweled version using 4,600 real rubies set in pavé. Surely, the most expensive shoes in history, and not even fit to be worn!

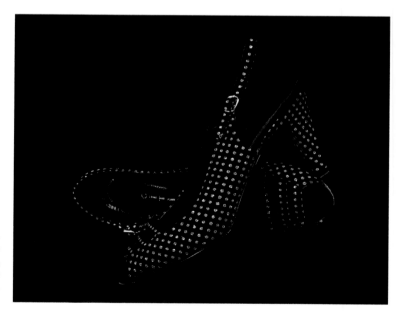

Twinkle, twinkle little stars. Glamorous slingbacks in stone-studded black velvet by Cities, circa 1975. *Courtesy of Cheap Thrills.* Value: $25-35.

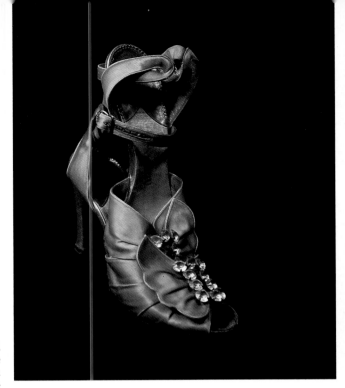

You'll dance until dawn in these glowing glacé satin slippers; from The Rollins Co., circa 1935. *Courtesy of Vintage Silhouettes.* Value: $45-65.

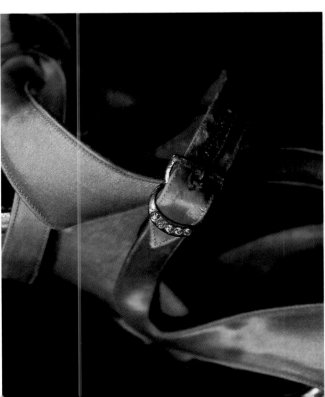

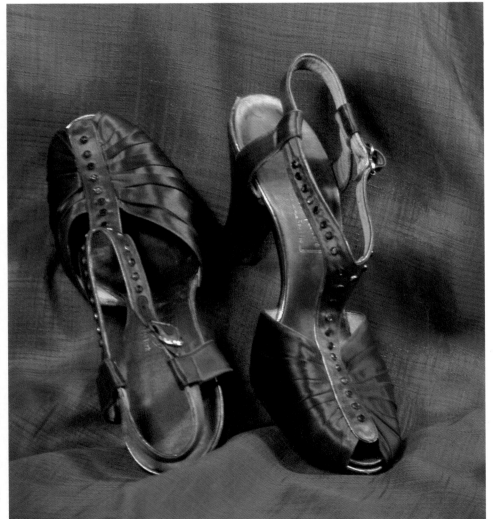

Dance slippers strap on with rhinestone razzle-dazzle; by I. Miller, circa 1935. Value: 95-115. *Courtesy of Lindy's Shoppe.*

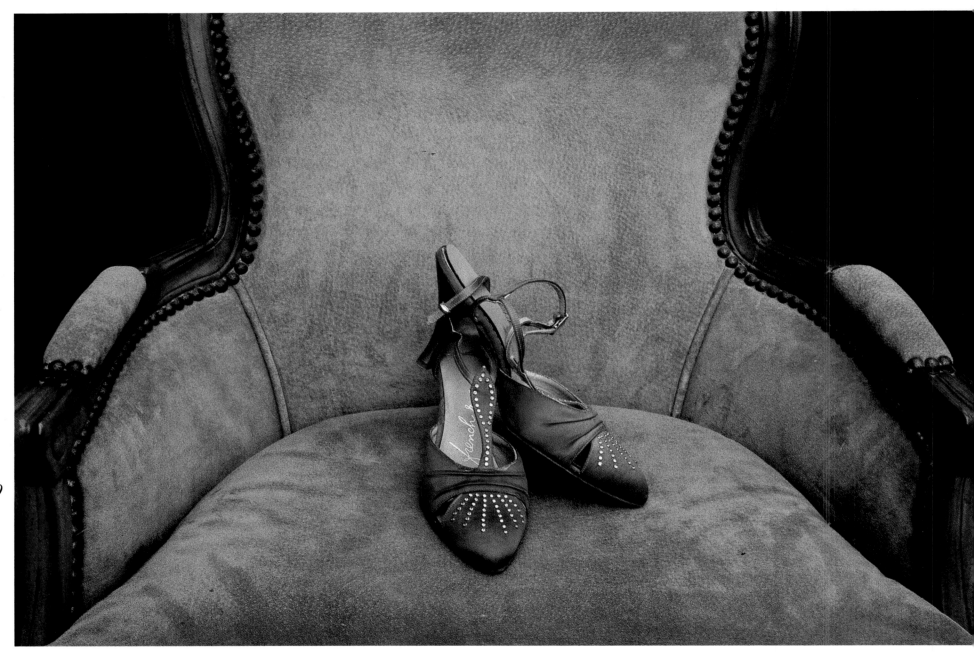

A starburst of rhinestones on sky-blue satin evening pumps from
Chandler's, circa 1959. *Courtesy of Lindy's Shoppe.* Value: $55-75.

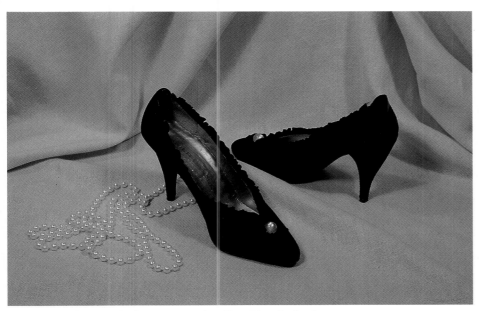

A pearl on suede dress pumps that flirt with a froth of satin ruffles at the throat. From the Paris salon of Xavier Danaud. *Courtesy of Lottie Ballou.* Value: $55-75.

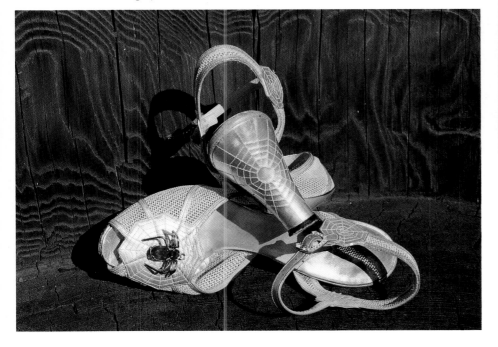

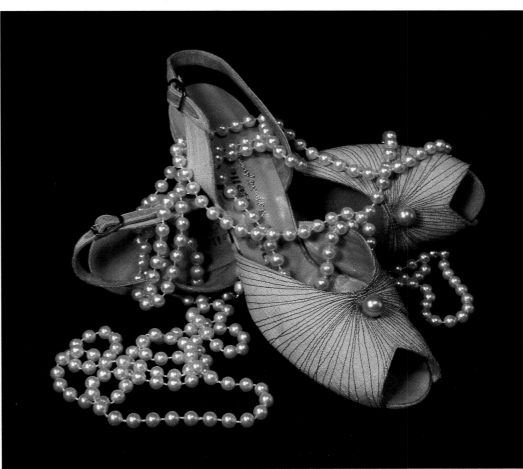

Above: Topstitch tendrils fan out from a perfect pearl on a bed of ivory silk; from Andrew Geller, circa 1939. *Courtesy of Luxe.* Value: $55-75.

Left: An important pair of sandals by Delman. These shoes exhibit extraordinary workmanship, including the webbing, which is outlined on silver kid heels. The "ruby" and silver spiders are pins that may be removed from the vamps to be worn on a bodice, by the less daring customer. This innovative design may be attributed to Roger Vivier, who worked for Delman in 1937 (and again, exclusively, in 1940–41 and 1945–47). If so, then the surrealistic theme is especially interesting, since we know Vivier's sketches for a raft-soled shoe were rejected by Delman, only to show up in Schiaparelli's collection of 1938. Perhaps there was an exchange of ideas between these two great designers? *Collection of Cynde Grossman.* Value: $165-195.

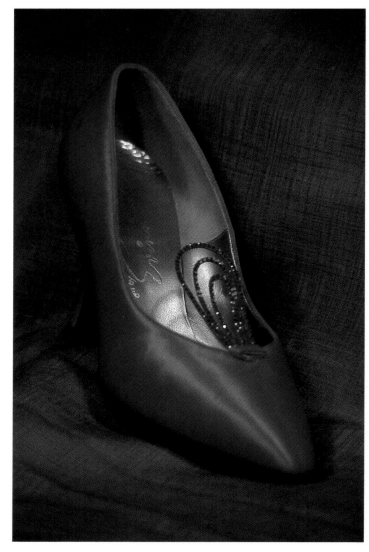

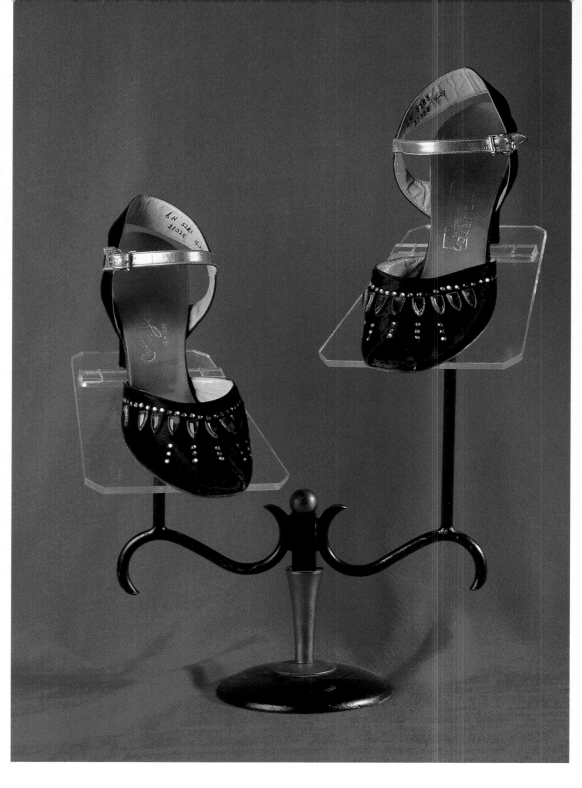

Above: Mock rubies leap like a flame at the throat of these satin pumps from the early 1960s. *Courtesy of Luxe.* Value: $45-65.

Right: A winning pair of party shoes by Jon Burton, bejeweled in the *rouge et noir* of roulette for a lucky lady in 1930. *Courtesy of Lindy's Shoppe.* Value: $95-115.

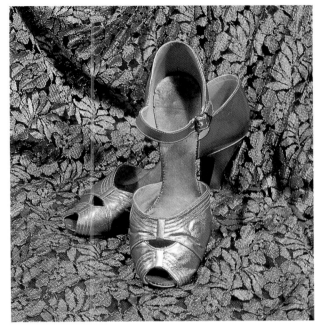

Gold kid T-straps on a sturdy heel were ideal for the Charleston. The style was first designed by André Perugia in the early 1920s to keep shoes firmly strapped to the feet of his high-kicking customers. *Courtesy of It's About Time.* Value: $35-55.

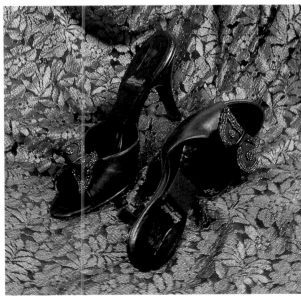
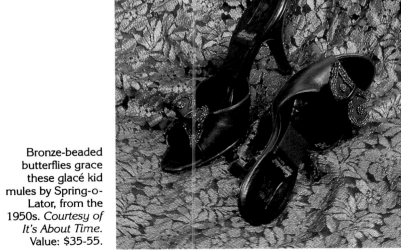

Bronze-beaded butterflies grace these glacé kid mules by Spring-o-Lator, from the 1950s. *Courtesy of It's About Time.* Value: $35-55.

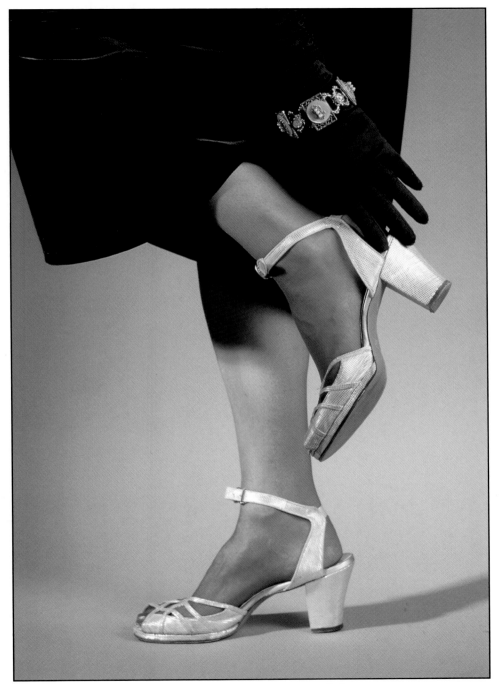

103

Ankle-strap silver platform sandals from the 1940s, aptly labeled "Cinderella." *Collection of Sheryl Birkner.* Value: Special.

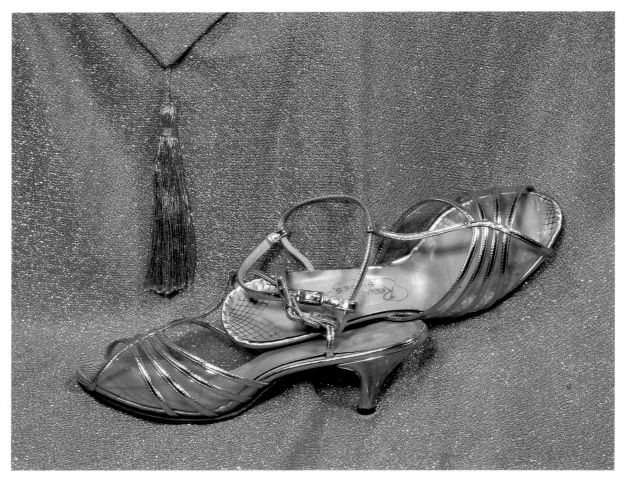

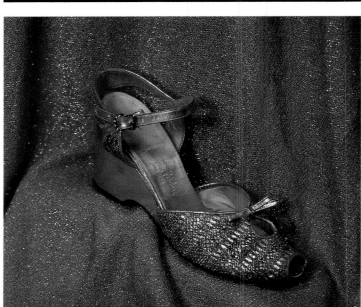

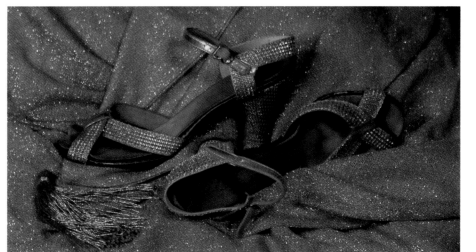

Above left: The ubiquitous strippy sandal in gold kid, a touch of glamour at suburban cocktail parties and other "little evenings," circa 1959. This pair is from Reeves, a national chain store located on the main street of most towns in that era. *Courtesy of Lottie Ballou.* Value: $15-25.

Above right: Silver lamé for heel and toe on a wedge of silver kid. Designed by Sommer & Kaufman in the mid-1940s. *Courtesy of Barbara Grigg Vintage Fashion.* Value: $45-65.

Left: Strips of gold lamé give the appearance of woven metal, forming cross-banded sandals from the late 1930s. *Courtesy of Vintage Silhouettes.* Value: $45-65.

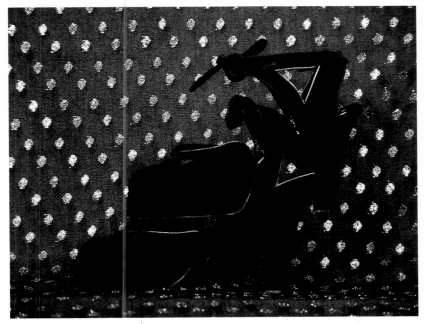

The mix of black satin or suede, with gold or silver kid, was popular for evening circa 1935. From I. Miller, a topstitched ankle strap. *Collection of Laurie Gordon.* A broad single-bar shoe by G. H. Baker slips inside. *Courtesy of Vintage Silhouettes .*Value: Special.

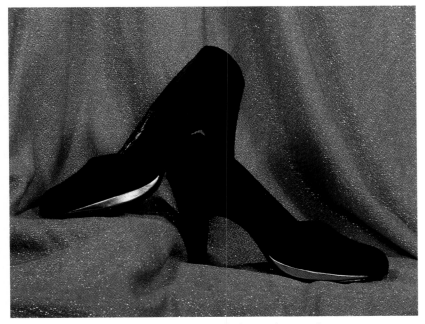

Black moiré shimmers softly and gold kid lights each step of these sophisticated-lady pumps. By I. Miller, circa 1945. *Courtesy of Barbara Grigg Vintage Fashion.* Value: $65-95.

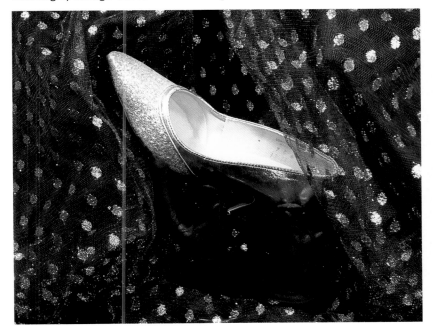

All that glitters is gold in a pair of stiletto dress pumps from the mid-1960s. *Courtesy of It's About Time.* Value: $15-25.

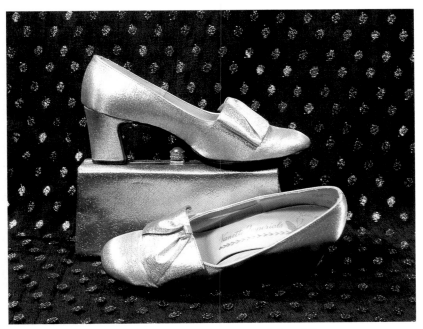

Broad of heel and bold of bow, pumps in man-made lamé the color of fire-lit champagne. This is early 1970s style on its best behavior. *Courtesy of It's About Time.* Value: $15-25.

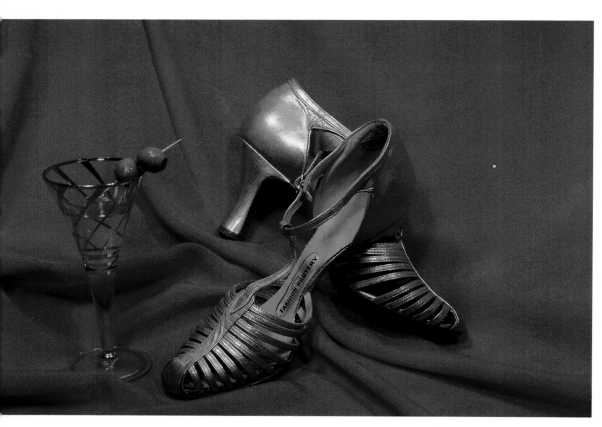

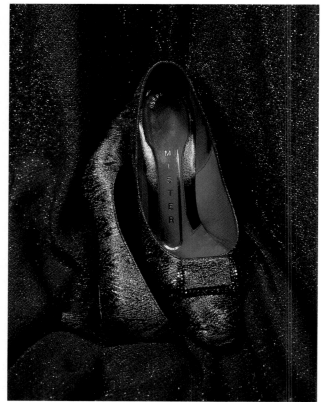

Above: Bottoms up, silver kid dance shoes are as classic as a martini. By Fashion Bootery, from the late 1920s or early 1930s. *Courtesy of Lottie Ballou.* Value: $45-65.

Right: A bevy of silver slippers in ankle-strap and T-strap, suitable for dancing under the stars of 1925. Left: From Carlson's department store in Grant Falls; Center: from Qualicraft. *Left shoe courtesy of Vintage Silhouettes; others courtesy of Lindy's Shoppe.* Value: $55-75.

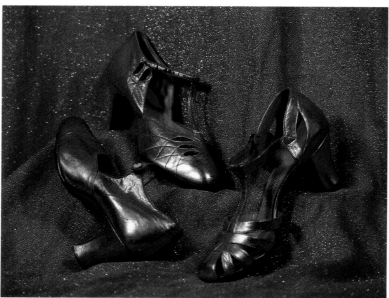

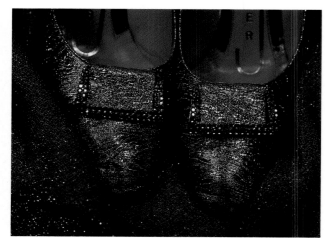

Above two: These court shoes feature buckles rimmed with iridescent rhinestones. These are the Mister J label from Joseph Magnin, circa 1967. *Courtesy of Cheap Thrills.* Value: $25-35.

The Feminine Foot

If you enjoy being a girl, then shoes are a natural form of self-expression. In rainbow colors of kid and suede, with flirty bows. In crisp linen embroidered with daisies, or smooth silk strewn with roses. The boudoir is another favorite province of femininity, whether your taste runs to quilted satin for comfort or marabou for glamour.

BOWS ON HER TOES

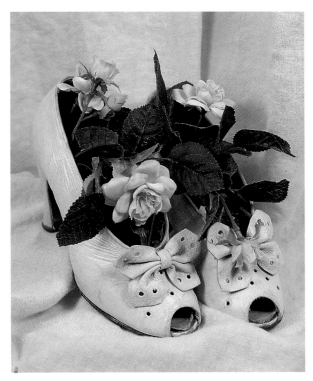

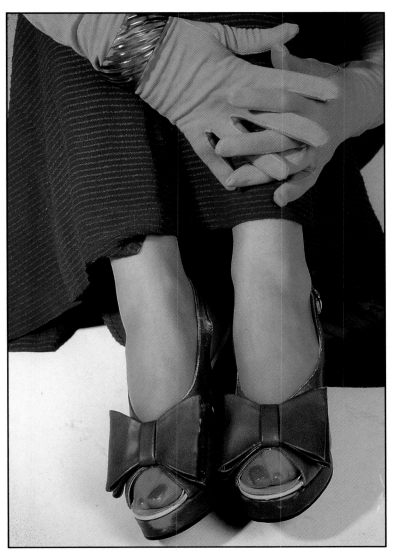

Above right: The sweetest silhouette of the 1930s in peep-toe pumps, shaped from white kid then tied like a candy box with perforated bows; by RoyalCraft. *Collection of Sylvia and Richard Unger.* Value: Special.

Right: Romantic sandals by Dominic Romano, ideal for dancing the night away in a chiffon ball gown, circa 1950. In pearlized pink kid, with a pearl cluster knotting each self-bow. *Collection of Connie Beers.* Value: Special.

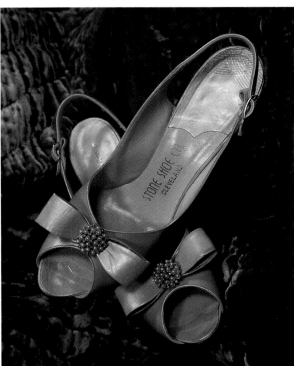

Big flat bows make a bold fashion statement on spring-green platform sandals by Patinos, circa 1945. *Collection of Viola de Cou.* Value: Special.

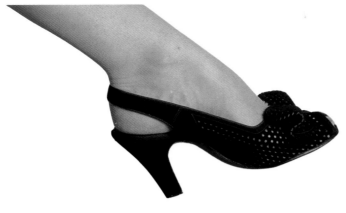

Plump bow graces the peep-toe of this perforated suede slingback in chocolate. Designed circa 1949 by Palter De Liso for De Liso Debs. *Collection of Pamela Joyce.* Value: Special.

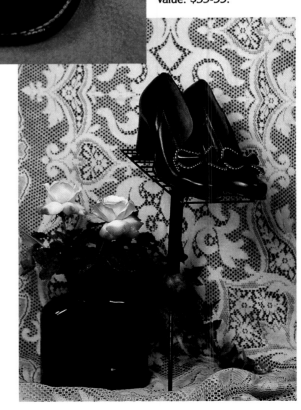

White kid whipcords around a pleated black kid bow, typical of the fine detailing to be found on Red Cross shoes from the mid-1930s. This was before the label became associated with sensible styling for women of a certain age, in the mid-1960s. *Author's collection.* Value: $35-55.

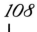

Double your pleasure, with rolled and ruffled self-bows on black kid peek-a-boo pumps, by Flint & Kent, circa 1950. Courtesy of Lottie Ballou. Value: $35-55.

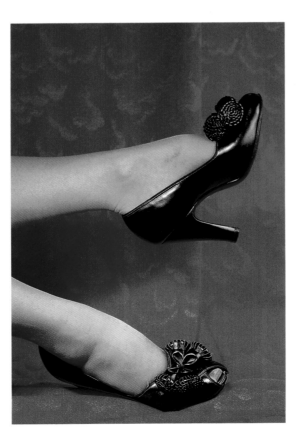

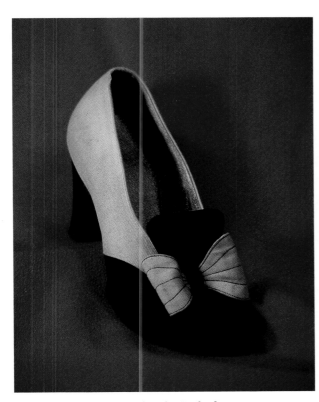

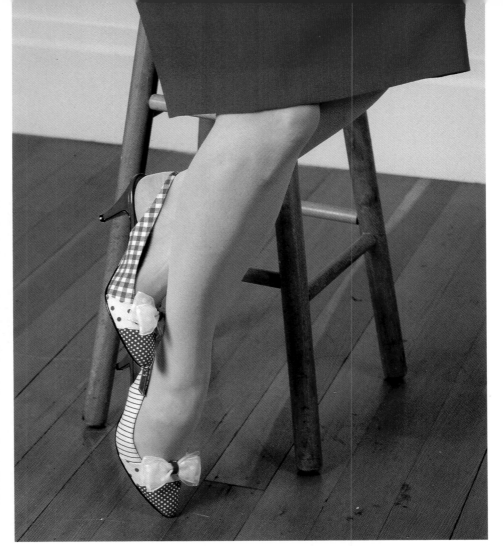

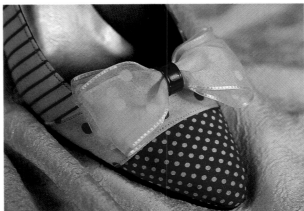

This lovely shoe is a lonely single. Its mate was actually stolen from a vintage clothing dealer in Northern California. It is easy to see why this petite shoe was such an object of desire, with its saucy bow and true-blue coloring. From the 1930s shoe salon in Ransohoff's of San Francisco. *Courtesy of The Blue Parrot.* Value: Special.

Darling slingbacks from De Liso Debs, circa 1965. Gingham and polka dots mix like a recipe for cherry cobbler, with the added fillip of a sugar-white bow. *Author's collection.* Value: $25-45.

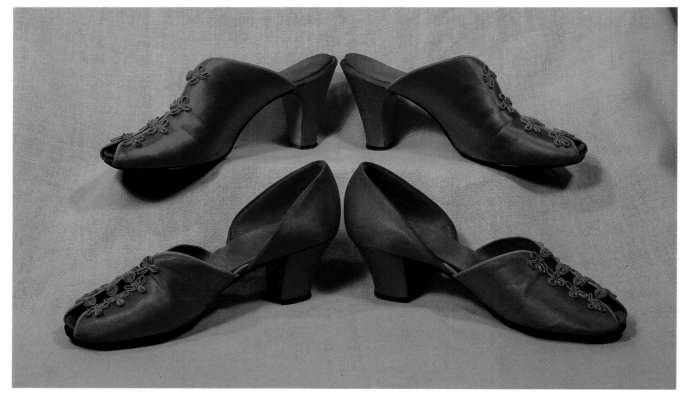

These slippers share the same color, trim, and label. But they were clearly designed for different functions during the style-conscious 1930s. Wear the high-heeled mules by Daniel Green with a satin robe for hostessing. Then slip on the low-heeled version by his Comfies label for breakfasting. *Courtesy of Lottie Ballou.* Value: $35-55.

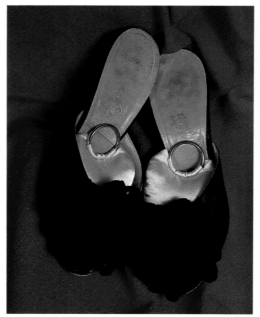

What a darling pair of mules in sapphire satin with peep-toe pompoms. These are from the I. Magnin shoe salon, circa 1960. *Collection of Connie Beers.* Value: Special.

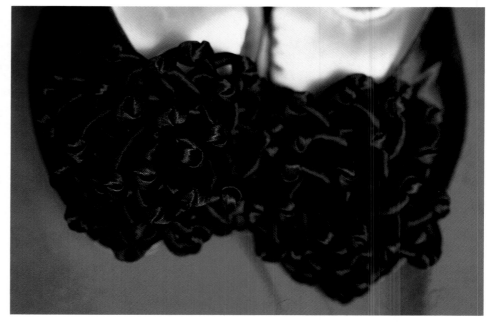

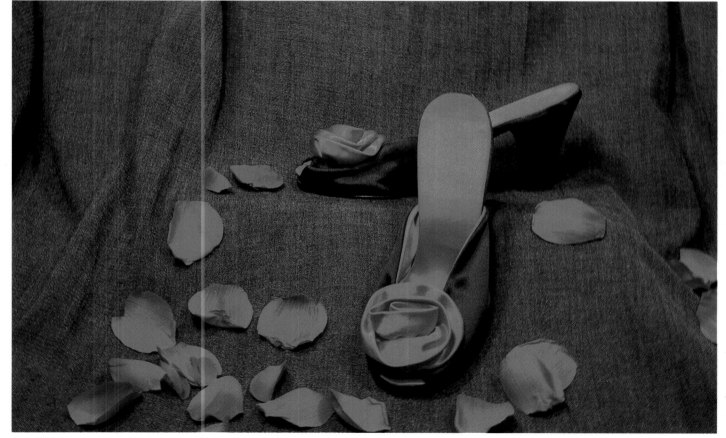

Walk in satin as soft as rose petals, in these black and red mules from the 1950s. *Courtesy of Lottie Ballou.* Value: $25-35.

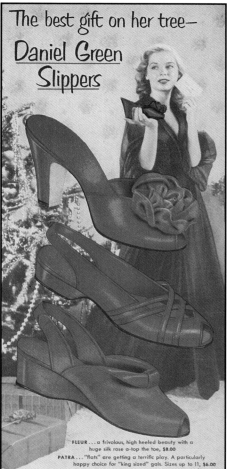

The best gift on her tree—
Daniel Green
Slippers

FLEUR...a frivolous, high heeled beauty with a huge silk rose a-top the toe, $8.00
PATRA..."flats" are getting a terrific play. A particularly happy choice for "king sized" gals. Sizes up to 11, $6.00
BONNY...for the lass who likes sweet simplicity and a

For Christmas 1951, Daniel Green said its comfy slippers would be "the best gift on her tree." And why not, when they were priced at $6 or $8 and came "in such dress-up colors as black, red, royal blue, and wine." We hope Santa will bring *Fleur* ! This is "a frivolous, high-heeled beauty with a huge silk rose atop the toe."

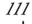

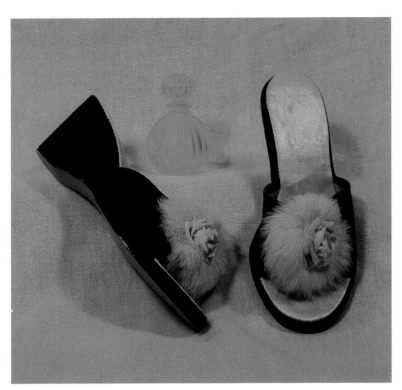

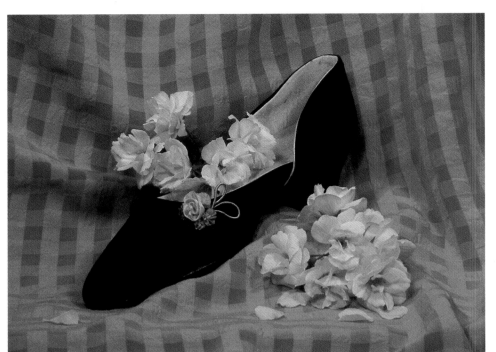

More roses for toes, a slipper from The Bootery, circa 1950. *Collection of Laurie Gordon.* Value: Special.

A puffball of rabbit fur dyed powder-puff pink lends feminine charm to a cozy pair of slippers, circa 1950. *Courtesy of Lottie Ballou.* Value: $15-25.

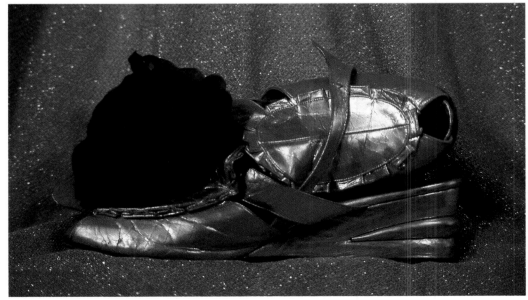

Silver kid is ruffled for the toe, pleated for the wedgie heel, in hostess slippers from the mid 1940s. *Courtesy of Barbara Grigg Vintage Fashion.* Value: $25-35.

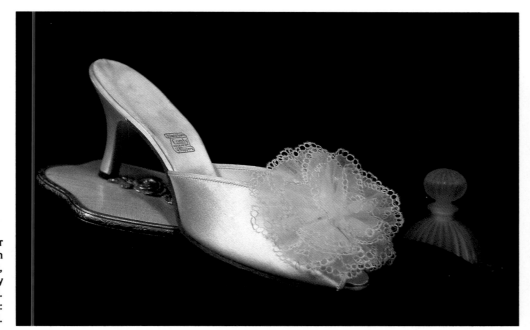

The classic boudoir slipper in white satin with a froth of lingerie lace and net, from the Comfy label by Daniel Green, circa 1965. *Author's collection.* Value: $15-25.

Initially, the backless slipper or mule was reserved for at-home wear. As with the pair shown here in black satin, ruffled with lamé kid, the mule was adorned with the most flirtatious trim of the shoemaker's art. These date to the early 1930s, and are labeled "Hostess Mules by H. Liebes & Co., San Francisco." *Collection of Laurie Gordon.* Value: Special.

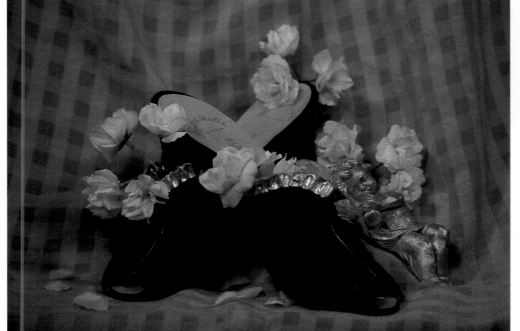

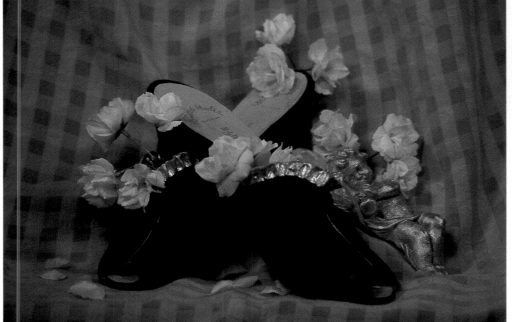

To the Victorians, embroidered slippers were considered a suitable yet personal gift from the hand of a young woman to her affianced. In that era, slippers were embued with the virtues of hearth, home, and faithfulness. The handwork shown was stitched in a man's size on a black velvet blank and was meant to be shaped by a cobbler as the upper part of a kid-soled slipper. *Collection of Carol Sidlow.* Value: Special.

113

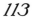

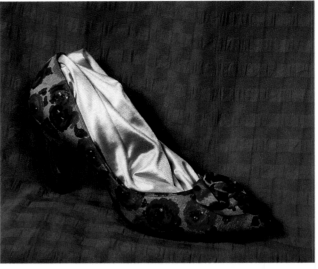

The lady won't be blue when she has these rhinestone-sparkled roses at her feet. Spikes from the mid-1960s, by Gaymode. *Courtesy of Lottie Ballou.* Value: $15-25.

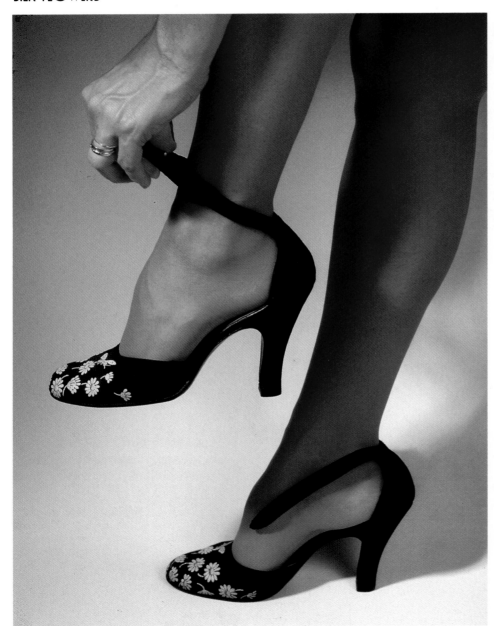

Black linen spike-heeled pumps with cut-away sides. The vamp is a sweet springtime scene, with hand-painted flowers and pert butterfly. This style is a perennial, but the leather soles and other construction techniques date these shoes to the early 1950s. *Courtesy of Lottie Ballou.* Value: $65-85.

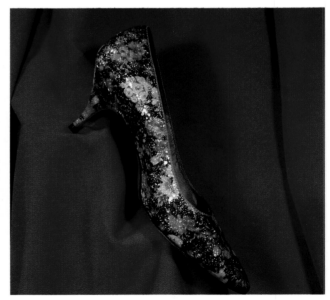

Low-heeled pumps, sprinkled with fairy dust for a night of magic in the late 1960s. By Kannauser of Palm Beach. *Courtesy of Cheap Thrills.* Value: $15-25.

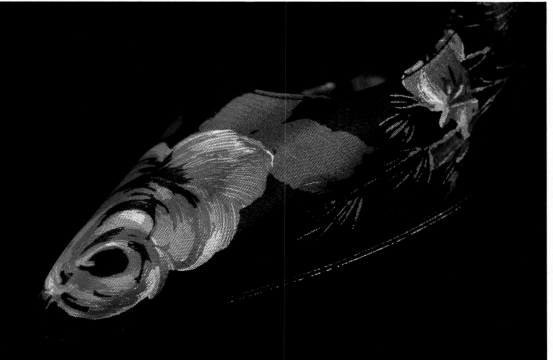

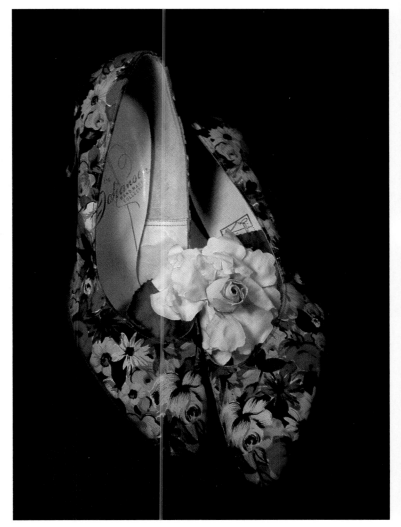

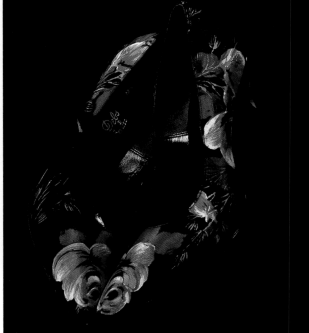

Above & Left: Palter De Liso shows his craft in these hand-screened silk pumps for De Liso Debs in the early 1960s. *Author's collection.* Value: $35-55.

Silkscreened tropical blooms make a lovely pair of pumps, circa 1960 by Johanssen's Handmade Collection. *Courtesy of It's About Time.* Value: $15-25.

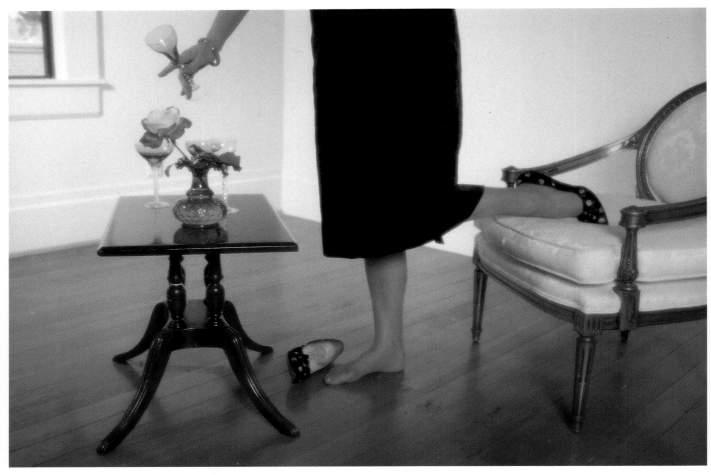

The ultimate rose-print black silk pump by Israel Miller for I. Magnin, circa 1960. *Courtesy of Lindy's Shoppe.* Value: $35-65.

Pucci-inspired print pumps by SRO, circa 1969. *Courtesy of The Blue Parrot.* Value: $15-25.

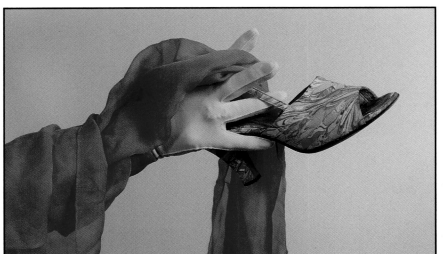

A wild psychedelic print is tamed by the conservative style of this slingback sandal by J. W. Robbins, circa 1962. *Courtesy of Lindy's Shoppe.* Value: $15-25.

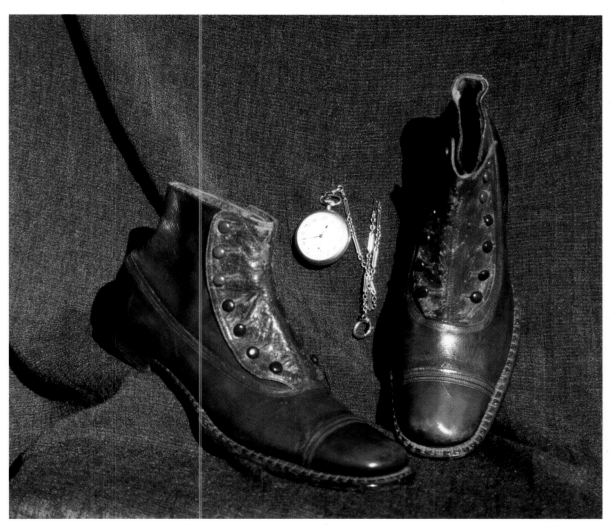

A fabulous find! These dress boots button on parallel tracks from instep to ankle, and with their slightly "bulldog" toes date to the Edwardian Era. They are part of the personal collection of Julia Bellacove, owner of The Blue Parrot in Roseville, California. She specializes in new\old stock but really can't pass up any pair of finely-crafted men's shoes.

Special Interests

FOR MEN ONLY

In the teens and early '20s, men favored the Bulldog style of high-button shoes, in polished tan calfskin. So named for the deep, squared toes that somewhat resembled the solid set of a Bulldog's jaw. These shoes were machine-made, thus readily available and affordable. Since they were also comfortable, they enjoyed a long popularity.

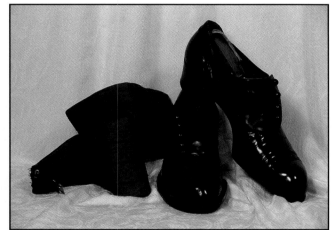

The *de rigeur* low-button dress shoe for a gentleman of the early 1920s, in black patent and gray kid. These are new\old stock, manufactured by the Reeves Shoe Co. and sold through The Florsheim Shop. Courtesy of The Blue Parrot. Value: Special.

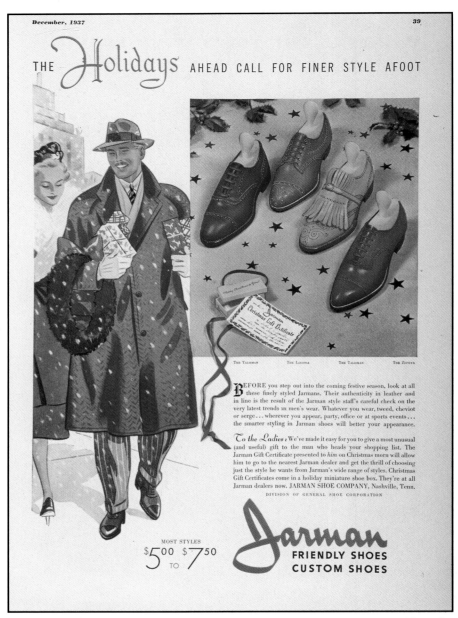

THE *Holidays* AHEAD CALL FOR FINER STYLE AFOOT

THE TALISMAN   THE LIVONIA   THE TALISMAN   THE ZEPHYR

BEFORE you step out into the coming festive season, look at all these finely styled Jarmans. Their authenticity in leather and in line is the result of the Jarman style staff's careful check on the very latest trends in men's wear. Whatever you wear, tweed, cheviot or serge . . . wherever you appear, party, office or at sports events . . . the smarter styling in Jarman shoes will better your appearance.

To the Ladies: We've made it easy for you to give a most unusual (and useful) gift to the man who heads your shopping list. The Jarman Gift Certificate presented to *him* on Christmas morn will allow him to go to the nearest Jarman dealer and get the thrill of choosing just the style he wants from Jarman's wide range of styles. Christmas Gift Certificates come in a holiday miniature shoe box. They're at all Jarman dealers now. JARMAN SHOE COMPANY, Nashville, Tenn.

DIVISION OF GENERAL SHOE CORPORATION

MOST STYLES
$5⁰⁰ TO $7⁵⁰

Jarman
FRIENDLY SHOES
CUSTOM SHOES

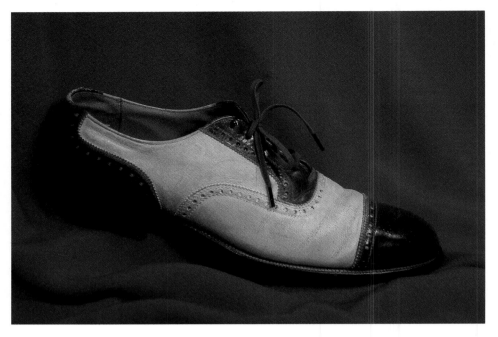

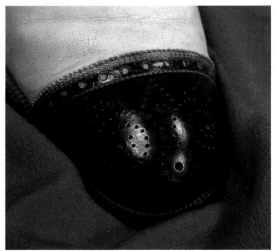

Classic and classy spectators from the early 1930s. The dress code of that day dictated a short season for these white and tan shoes, from Labor Day to Memorial Day. *Courtesy of It's About Time.* Value: $55-75.

A quartet of fine-grained kid brogues capture the soft amber glow of well-aged brandy. As advertised by Jarman in the December 1937 issue of *Esquire* magazine. The ad was geared to holiday shoppers. Since these shoes were priced at $5 to $7.50 a pair, they were luxury gifts in the waning years of the Depression. The company included a special note "to the ladies" who might otherwise hesitate to buy such a personal item: "We've made it easy for you to give a most unusual (and useful) gift to the man who heads your shopping list. The Jarman Gift Certificate presented to *him* on Christmas morn will allow *him* to go to the nearest Jarman dealer and get the thrill of choosing just the style he wants from Jarman's wide range of styles. Christmas Gift Certificates come in a holiday miniature shoe box."

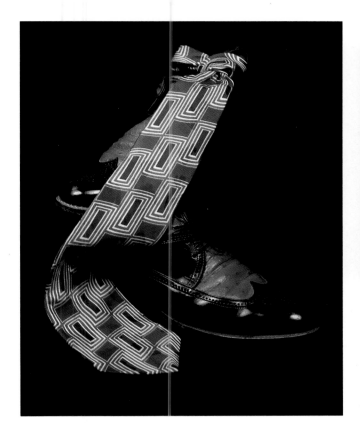

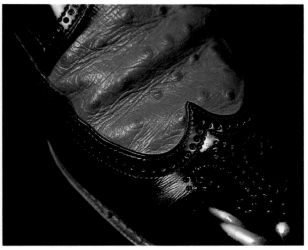

Walking right off the pages of Damon Runyon's *Guys & Dolls*, spectators with widow-peak wing-tips. Exotic leathers, such as the dyed ostrich shown here, were prized by natty dressers circa 1940. *Collection of Billy Jean Jones*. Value: Special.

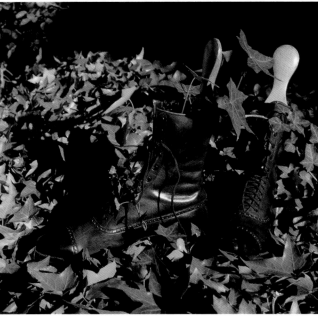

For the Ivy League, a fine pair of gray boots with perforated black tips. At the turn-of-the-century, men were inspired to sartorial splendor by Prince Edward. These boots were certainly custom-fitted, and may even have been ordered to match a bespoke gray flannel suit. *Courtesy of The Blue Parrot*. Value: Special.

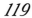

From Ivy League to "in the trenches." This is a much-worn work boot, circa 1939, a type that may have served as the model for soldiers' boots in World War II. *Courtesy of Lindy's Shoppe*. Value, the pair: $25-45.

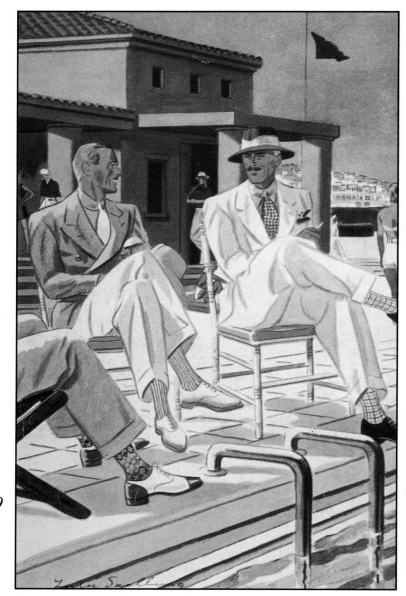

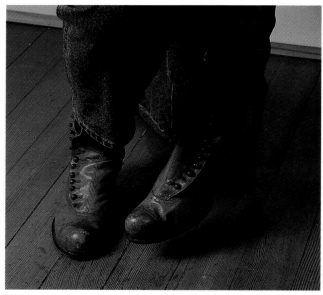

Sometimes we just can't resist borrowing from the boys, especially when it's a beautiful pair of vintage shoes in a smooth kid the color of cognac. Lindy Moore wears these "bulldog" high-button boots with her jeans and prairie skirts. Not that she overlooks the distaff side, though. "I just love shoes! I once bought out an entire shoe store, 600 pair of old\new stock. Don't ask me why, but if the shoe is for sale, I'll buy it." Lucky for us collectors, she also sells them at *Lindy's Shoppe* in Napa, California.

Interwoven socks in daring plaids, argyles, and stripes to set off the white linens of summer in this ad from the August 1934 issue of *Esquire*. The shoes are white buckskin, brown buckskin, and a spectator style in white buck and brown kid. Note the ties and jackets worn for lounging pool side, a far cry from today's casual dress code.

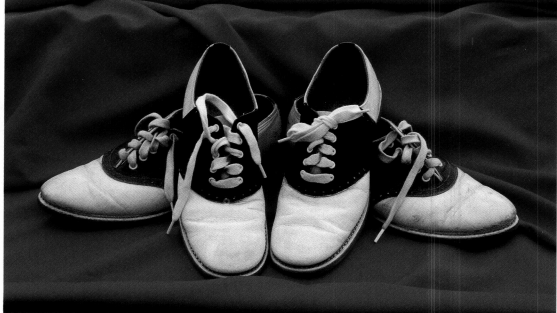

Saddle shoes are practically synonymous with the malt-shop crowd, given their extreme popularity with boppers and bobby-soxers. In 1949, Buster Brown offered thirty-seven variations on this enduring style. Both of these are by Spalding, for young men. *Courtesy of Lottie Ballou.* Value: $25-45.

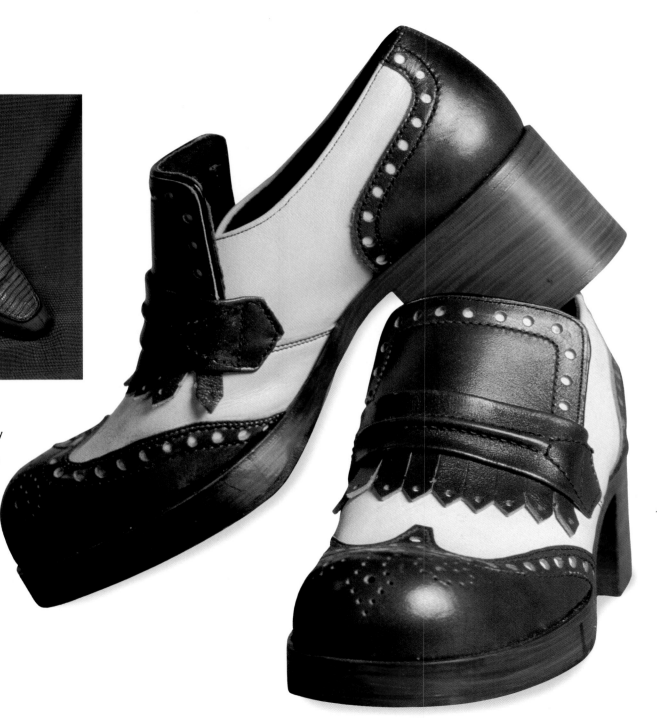

Above: Lounge-lizard loafers from the mid-60s. *Courtesy of It's About Time.* Value: $45-65.

Right: Keep on truckin' in new\old stock shoes by Roberts. They are from the mid-1970s and, like much clothing of that era, they are a polyglot. To the basic loafer silhouette add spectator color, platform heel, wing-tip toe, and kiltie vamp. *Courtesy of Lindy's Shoppe.* Value: $45-65.

THE WEDDING MARCH

In ancient Israel the transfer of a shoe could seal a bond or contract. It's just a short step in time to the wedding ritual of medieval Europe, whereby a bride's father passed her shoe to the groom, in symbol of marriage. Take one more leap forward, to the present-day custom of tying shoes to a newlywed's car for good luck.

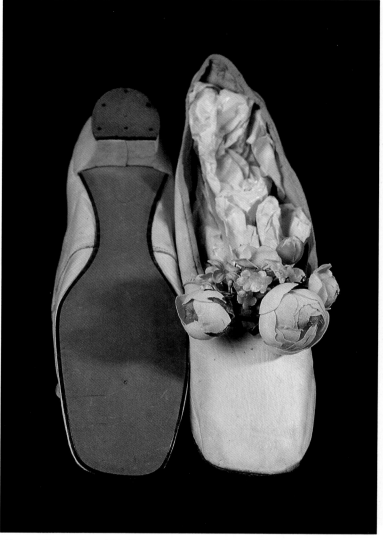

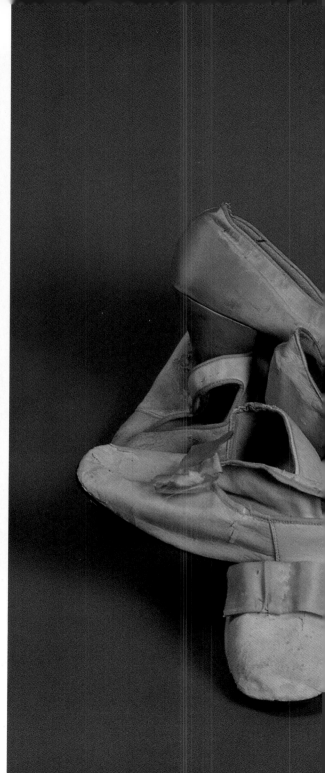

Above: These glove-kid slippers were worn at a wedding in 1889, the date meticulously recorded on the box in which they were lovingly tissue-wrapped and then passed down from mother to daughter. As can be seen by the barely-soiled soles, they are straights with no distinction between left and right. The original shoe clips had been removed, but no doubt the bride wore blossoms like the vintage silk roses shown here. *Courtesy of Lottie Ballou.* Value: Special.

Right: A bouquet in cream and white, silk and satin. These bridal shoes span several eras, but all convey the same message of sweet romance. *Courtesy of Lindy's Shoppe and Lottie Ballou.* Value: Special.

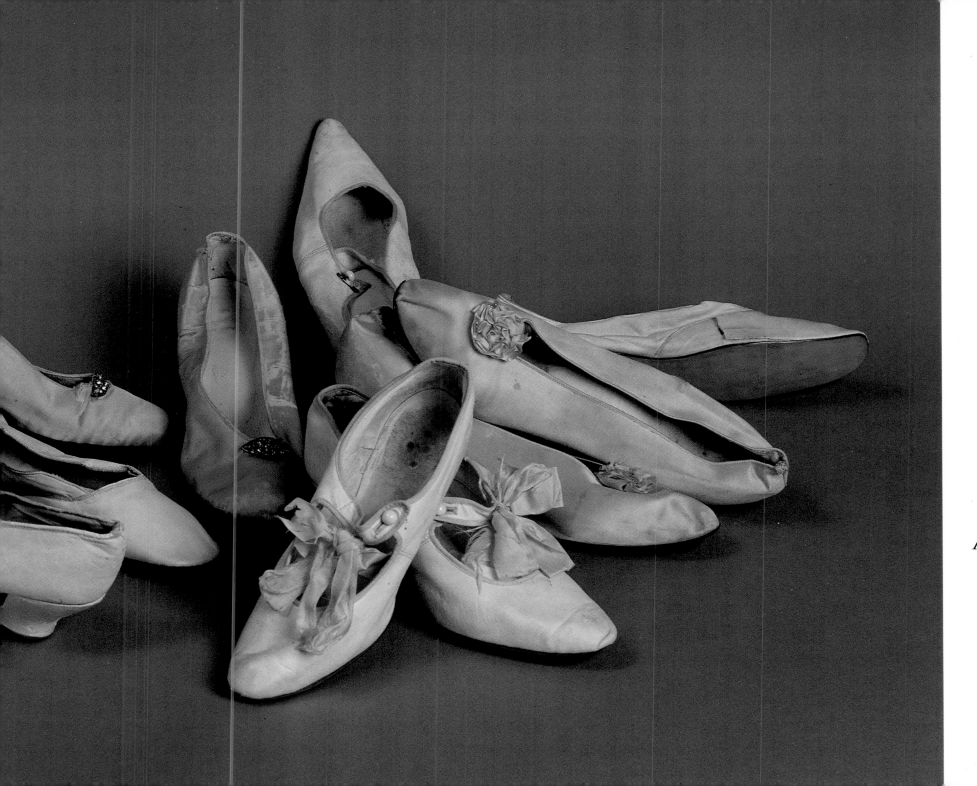

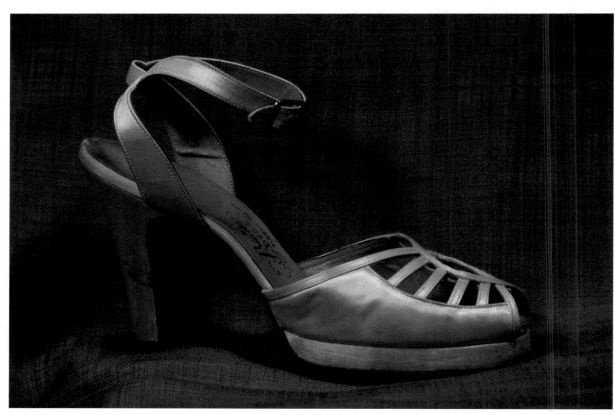

Wedding shoes for a wartime bride. She may have been married in a tailored gown, but her platform shoes are a tribute to the female form. *Collection of Laurie Gordon.* Value: Special.

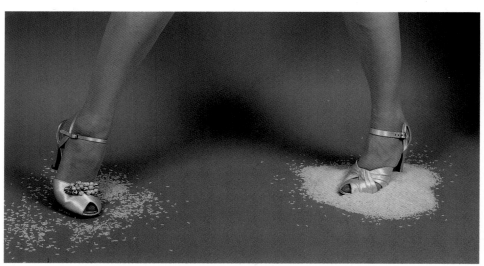

The traditional candlelight satin appears in an open-toe ankle strap, for a bride of the late 1930s or early 1940s (at right). *Collection of Laurie Gordon.* Compare this shoe to the ice blue satin ankle straps with pretty pearlized shoe clips, for a mother-of-the-bride, circa 1950. *Collection of Pamela Joyce.* Value (each): $45-65.

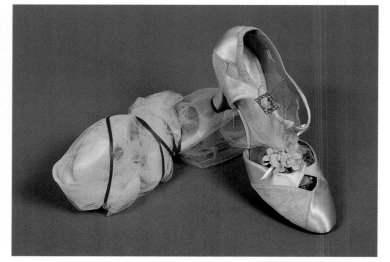

A flapper bride wore these satin T-straps with strass buckles, for a wedding day in the late 1920s. *Collection of Laurie Gordon.* Value: Special.

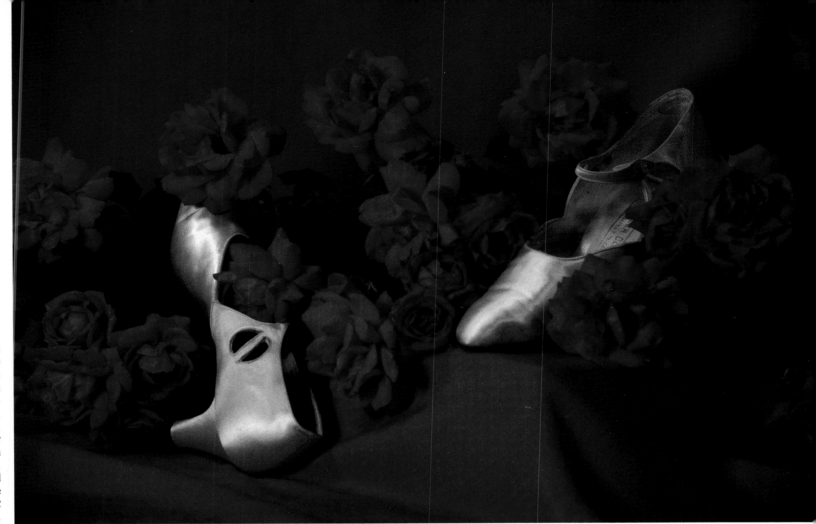

More satin bridal shoes from the 1920s, with peek-a-boo heels, peep out from a wedding bower. Although wedding shoes have sentimental value, much like children's, they are easier to come by. Presumably, brides wore their shoes but once and then carefully stored them away. Look for them in good condition, at reasonable prices. *Courtesy of Past Perfect.* Value: $65-85.

She got him today, he'll get her tonight! So the naughty saying goes, but in this case the bride was prepared. These black velvet slippers, aptly named *Oomphies*, were worn on a wedding night in the late 1940s. Perhaps, with a midnight-black lace negligee? *Courtesy of The Blue Parrot.* Value: Special.

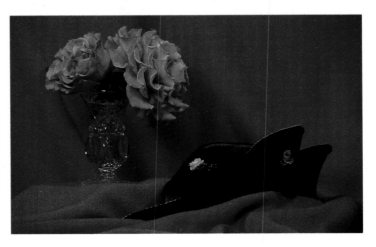

PATTER OF LITTLE FEET

Baby's first booty is an emblem of infancy. Whether bronzed or boxed or tied to the rear-view mirror, it is cherished as a keepsake from the first year of life. It is also symbolic of the passage into childhood, the toddling years when little feet move toward a widening horizon of exploration and development. For such reasons of sentiment, baby and children shoes are a favorite with collectors, even those who might not otherwise dabble in vintage fashion. Since wear and tear are the imprimatur of a busy and happy childhood, even somewhat frayed shoes are cherished.

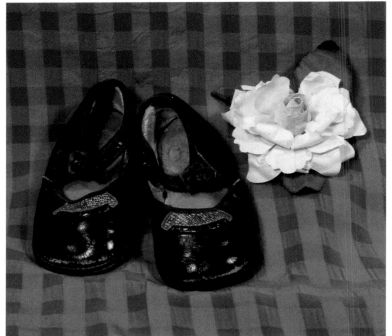

Do you remember your first party shoes? These perky patent Mary Janes were worn in 1945. *Collection of Carol Sidlow.* Value: Special.

126

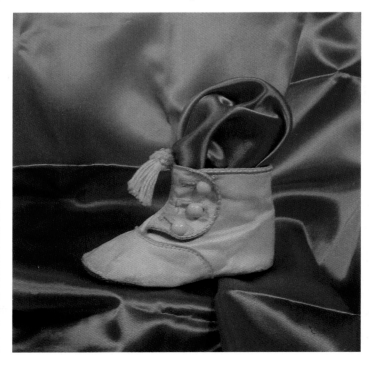

Who could miss baby's first step when she struts forth in these! Swish-swish goes the tassel of the white kid boot, circa 1915. *Courtesy of Rich Man, Poor Man.* Value: $55-75.

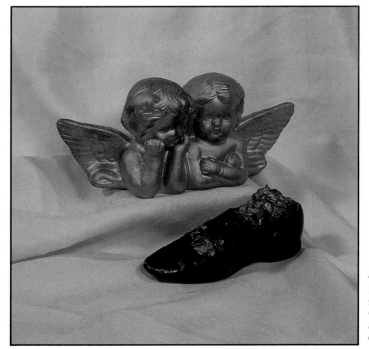

A single-bar dress pump in olive green glove-soft leather, circa 1910. *Collection of Violet de Coup.* Value: Special.

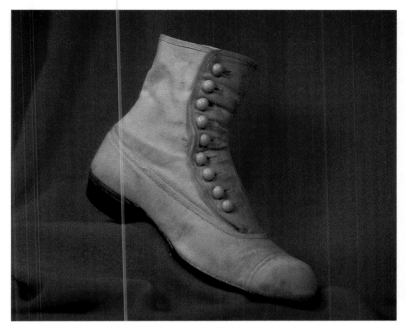

A young lady's high-button shoe, in cool white canvas for summer fun, circa 1915. Her little toes had plenty of room to wiggle in these fashionable bulldogs. The heel is of stacked wood, the buttons are of white glass. *Courtesy of The Blue Parrot.* Value: $115-125.

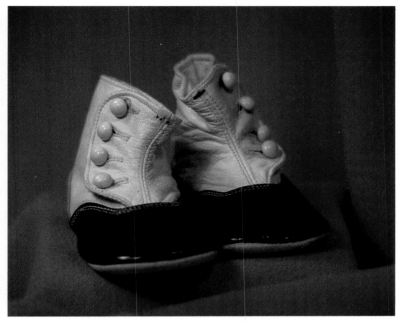

Dear little high-button boots, for the pride and joy of a Victorian mama. In shiny black patent and soft white kid, with four brilliant glass buttons. *Courtesy of The Blue Parrot.* Value: $95-115.

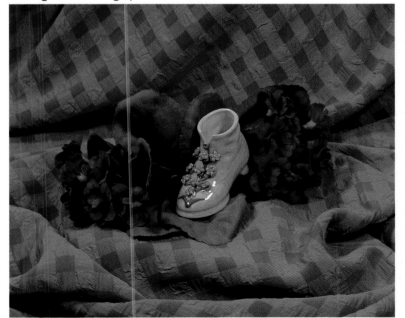

A shy pearlized white china booty with violet trim. Value: $15. *Courtesy of Rich Man, Poor Man.*

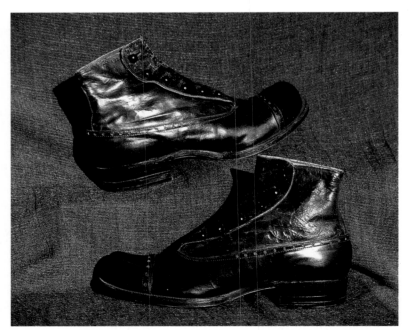

Children's shoes are often scuffed, but these Sunday-school brogues are visible proof of a young boy's best behavior. From the Edwardian era, when bulldog toes were also popular with grown-ups. *Courtesy of The Blue Parrot.* Value: $115-135.

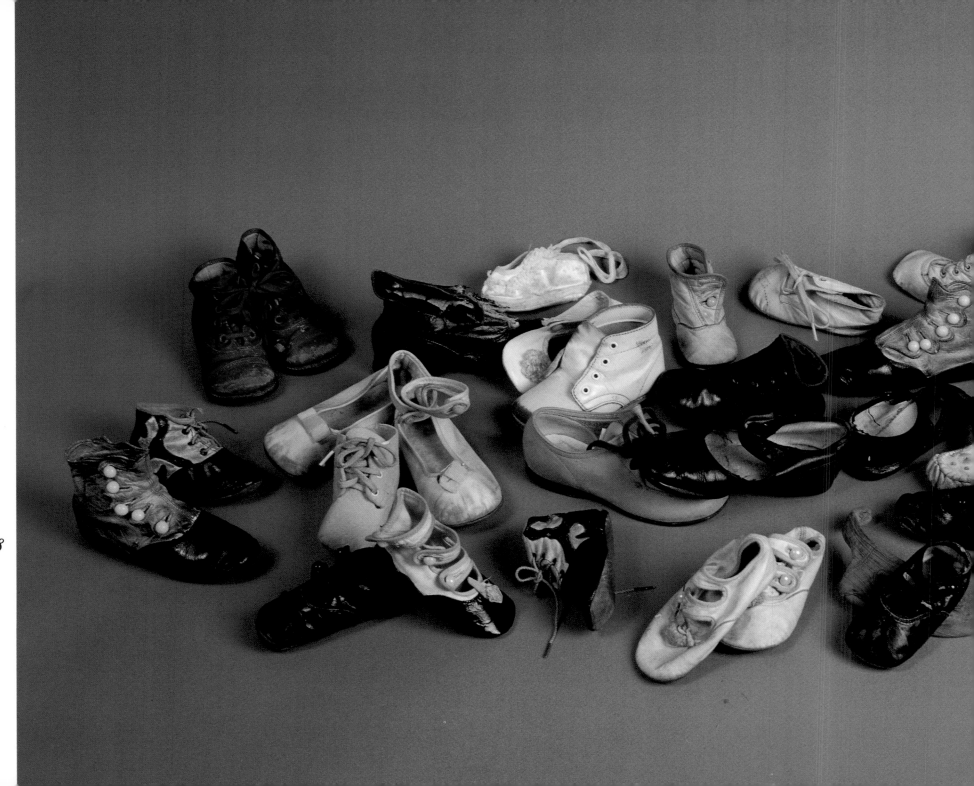

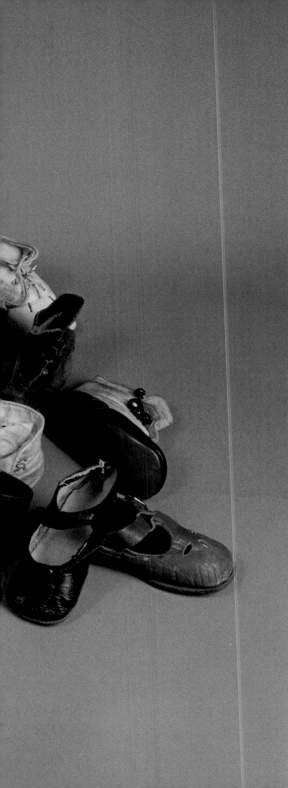

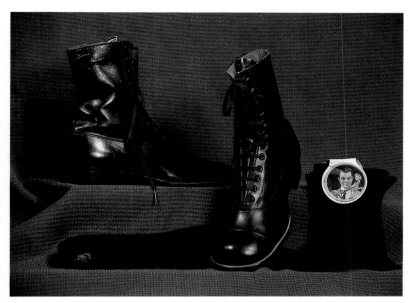

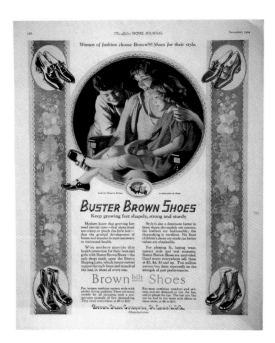

Buster Brown was the shoe of choice for boys in the 1920s. The quality of construction is evident in this pair of new\old stock boots in lustrous calfskin. Note the original display tag on the knee-high socks from the same era. *Courtesy of The Blue Parrot.* Value: boots, $125-135; socks, $25-45.

In this advertisement from the early 1920s, young mothers were urged to purchase Buster Brown shoes for their growing boys and girls.

129

For many collectors, children's shoes are all the more charming when they show the wear and tear of active playtime. This wonderful assortment runs the gamut, having been worn at various stages of childhood; circa 1900 to 1950. *Courtesy of Lindy's Shoppe.* Value: Special.

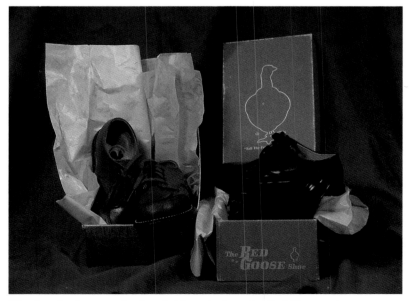

Shoebox fresh, two pair of new\old stock shoes by Red Goose, circa 1950. *Courtesy of The Blue Parrot.* Value (each pair): $45-65.

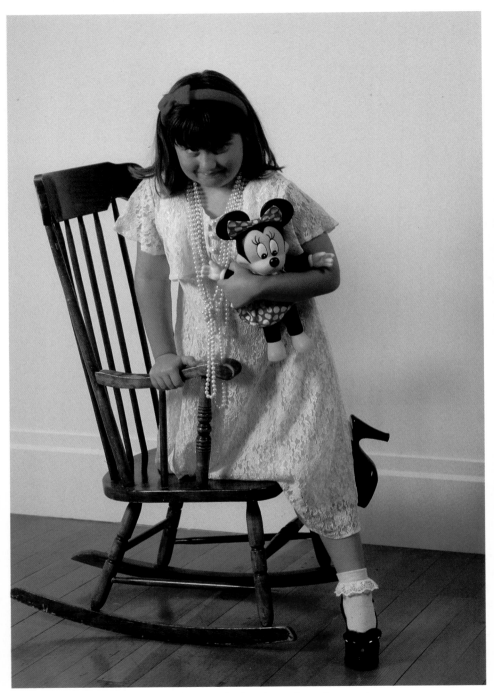

Jamie Lynn Saunders, the author's daughter, plays dress-up in platforms by Israel Miller salon, circa 1945. She's just seven years old in this photo, making the shoes her senior by fifty years.

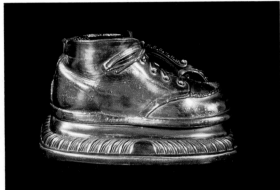

The sentimental practice of bronzing baby shoes began in the 1920s, and reached its apogee in the 1950s. Bronzed here, a sturdy oxford that was laced snugly on a little foot in the early 1950s. *Collection of Gail Pocock.* Value: Special.

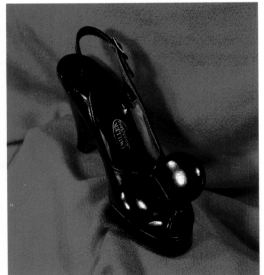

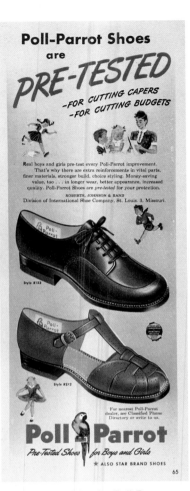

Poll-Parrot Shoes
are
PRE-TESTED
−FOR CUTTING CAPERS
−FOR CUTTING BUDGETS

Real boys and girls pre-test every Poll-Parrot improvement. That's why there are extra reinforcements in vital parts, finer materials, stronger build, choice styling. Money-saving value, too . . . in longer wear, better appearance, increased quality. Poll-Parrot Shoes are *pre-tested* for your protection.

ROBERTS, JOHNSON & RAND
Division of International Shoe Company, St. Louis 3, Missouri.

Style #133

Style #272

For nearest Poll-Parrot dealer, see Classified Phone Directory or write to us.

Poll Parrot
Pre-Tested Shoes for Boys and Girls
★ ALSO STAR BRAND SHOES

65

In the late 1930s, the Poll-Parrot company assured budget-conscious moms that its shoes "are pre-tested for your protection . . . (by) real boys and girls."

The same shoes by I. Miller in close-up. For Jamie, it's not the vintage lineage that counts, but the fact that these shoes bear an uncanny resemblance to a certain set of mouse ears!

Novelties

GARDEN PARTY

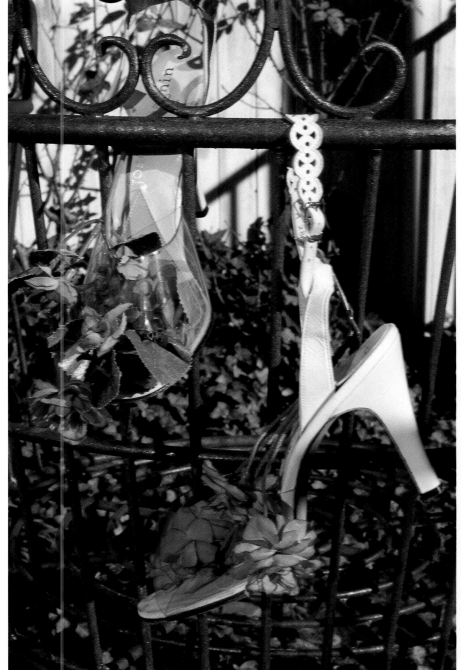

Cut like a garden trellis at the ankle strap, this creamy kid sandal with its self-proclaimed invisible vamp sold at the Joseph Magnin shoe salon, circa 1979. *Courtesy of Cheap Thrills.* Value: $15-25.

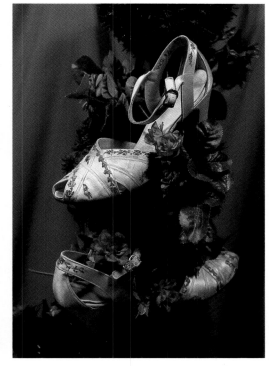

Left: Garlands of shy violets are hand-painted on dainty ivory kid ankle strap sandals, from the early 1930s. *Courtesy of Lottie Ballou.* Value: $55-75.

Below: Overall floral embroidery on linen, rivaling the glory of cherry blossoms in the spring. These sweet linen shoes are from the Desert Bootery in Palm Springs, circa 1979. *Courtesy of Barbara Grigg Vintage Fashion.* Value: $15-35.

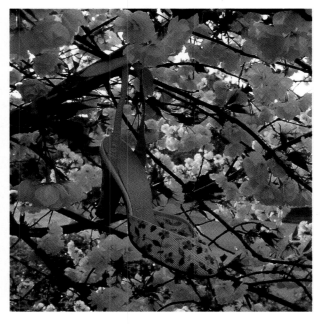

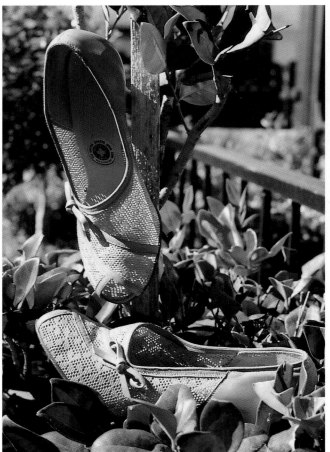

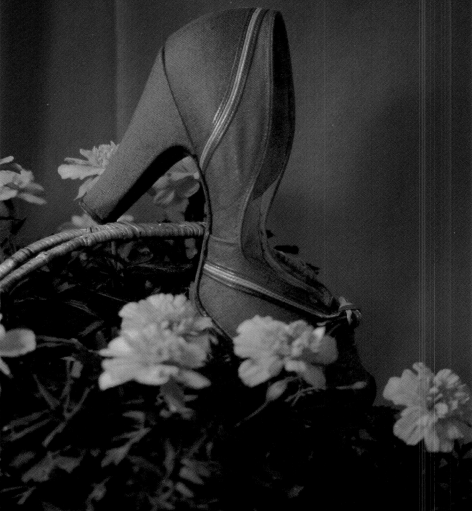

Above: Fall colors, falling into the potted marigolds. These décolleté pumps are by Roberta, circa 1955. *Courtesy of Lindy's Shoppe.* Value: $25-45.

Left: Red Cross mesh pumps with cutaway sides, in barely-there beige. These shoes would have been cool, comfortable, and chic for city streets in the mid-1930s. *Courtesy of C & L Antiques.* Value: $35-55.

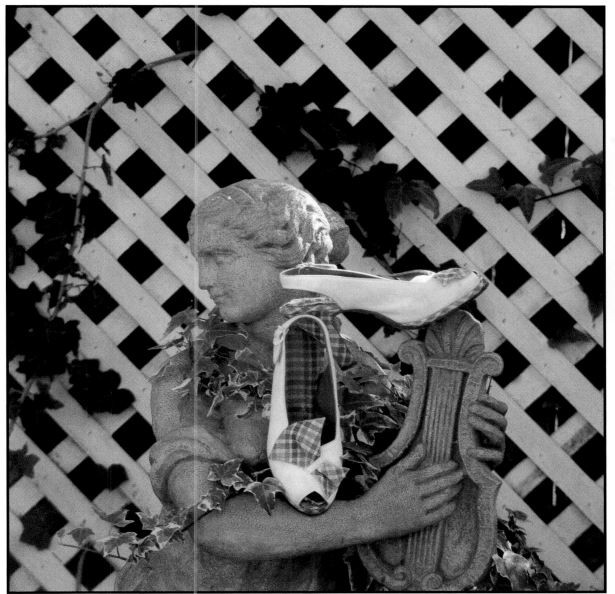

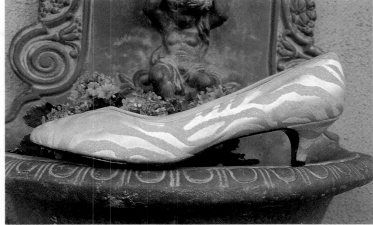

Above: Ivory satin pumps glitter with mock zebra stripes; by Imperial, circa 1969. *Courtesy of Cheap Thrills.* Value: $10-15.

Left: Graced by the perennial charm of gingham, these white suede platforms are timeless in their appeal. By John Morton, circa 1945. *Courtesy of Time After Time.* Value: $75-95.

133

FRUIT SALAD

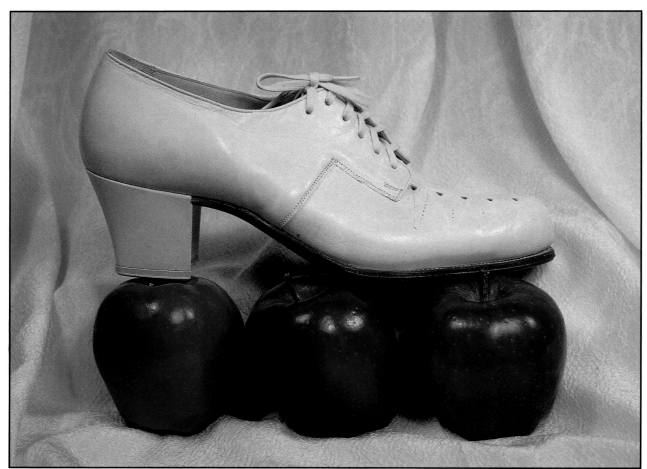

What to wear for summertime fun, circa 1935? Why, perforated open-toe kid oxfords, of course. From new\old stock, they boast a patented Flex-Spot arch support. *Courtesy of Luxe.* Value: $35-55.

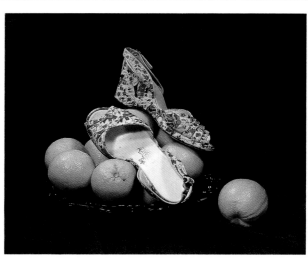

Print wedgies were typically worn with dirndl skirts or slacks, or perhaps the new play suits from Clare McCardell's sportswear line, circa 1950. *Courtesy of Lottie Ballou.* Value: $15-25.

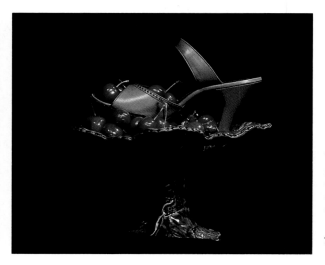

This stiletto mule in grape-green kid holds on tight, with its seeded straps. For hot summer nights circa 1979, by QualiCraft. *Author's collection.* Value: $10-25.

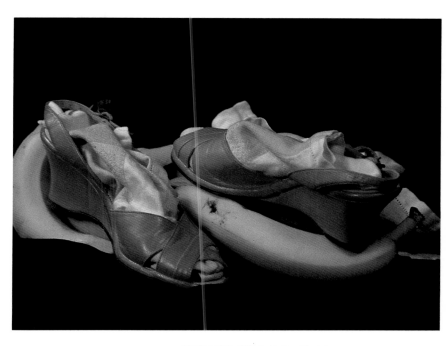

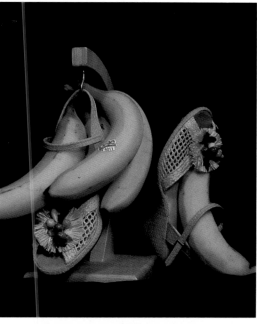

Above: From Joyce of California, circa 1955, a dusky orange wedge-heel sandal. *Courtesy of Luxe.* Value: $15-25.

Right: These new\old stock woven straw sandals are from the mid-1950s and feature the popular fruit-basket motif. *Courtesy of Lindy's Shoppe.* Value: $25-45.

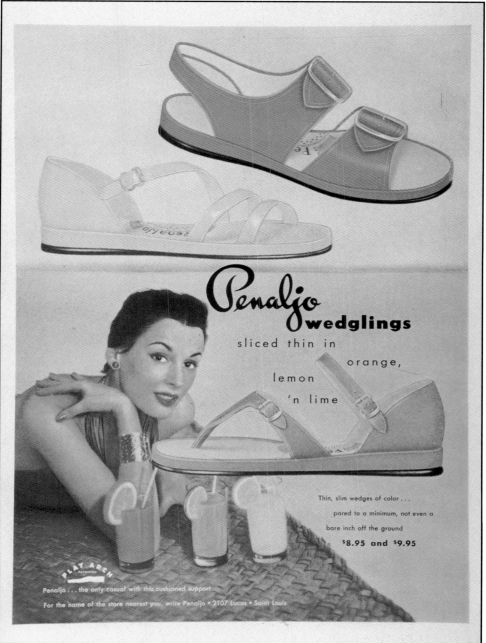

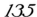

Penaljo **wedglings**

sliced thin in

orange,

lemon

'n lime

Thin, slim wedges of color . . .
pared to a minimum, not even a
bare inch off the ground

$8.95 and $9.95

PLAY ARCH PATENTED

Penaljo . . . the only casual with this cushioned support

For the name of the store nearest you, write Penaljo • 2107 Lucas • Saint Louis

135

Citrus colors are always cool for summer fashions. In April 1950, Penaljo advertised open-toed "wedglings . . . sliced thin in orange, lemon 'n lime."

The alligator bag was used by the author's mother in the early 1940s and it still garners compliments when used today. The alligator pumps are from the same era and make a perfect match. Value: bag, $55-75; pumps, $45-65.

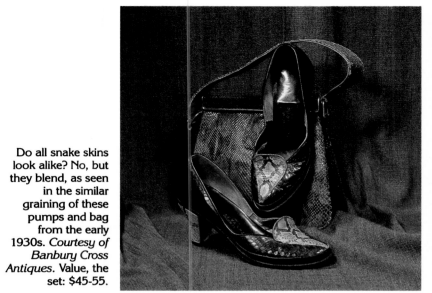

Do all snake skins look alike? No, but they blend, as seen in the similar graining of these pumps and bag from the early 1930s. *Courtesy of Banbury Cross Antiques.* Value, the set: $45-55.

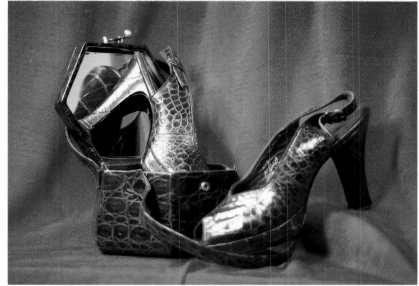

Chunky platforms reflect in the mirrored lid of a plump octagon bag, a double kiss of chocolate crocodile. Both are from Saks Fifth Avenue, circa 1945. *Courtesy of Luxe.* Value: shoes, $75-95; bag, $95-115.

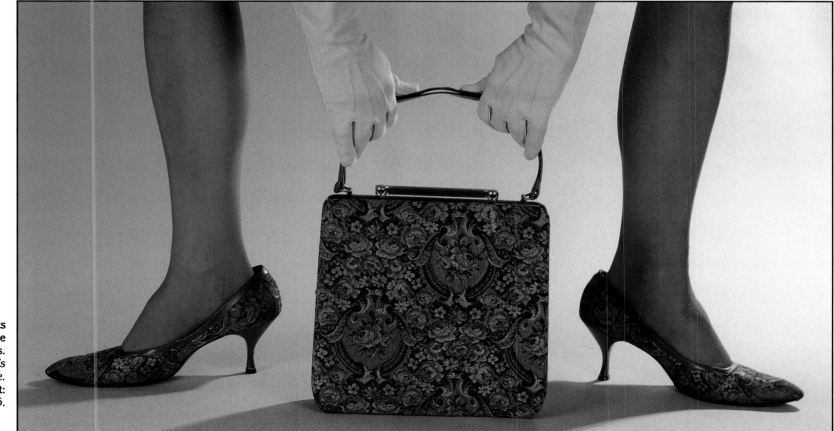

Tapestry sets were all the rage in the 1950s. *Courtesy of It's About Time.* Value, the set: $35-55.

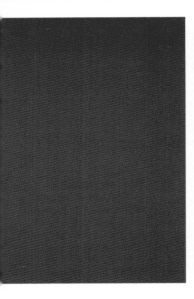

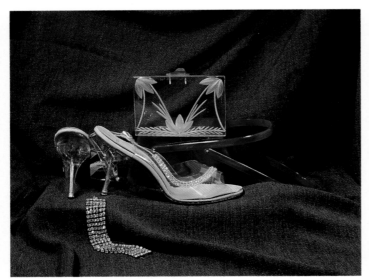

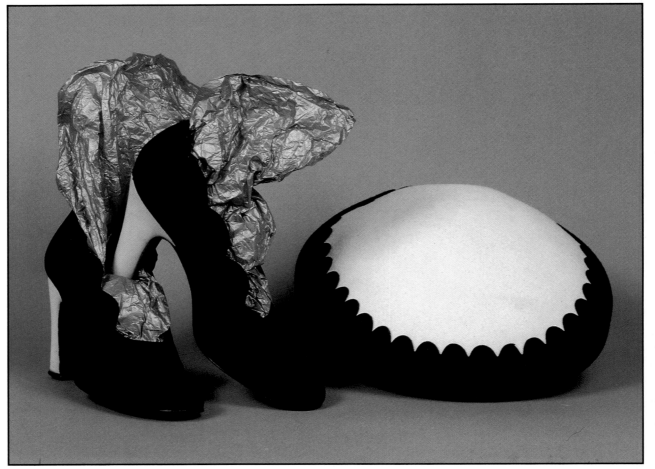

Above left: These shoes are well-matched to the boxy faux tortoise bag; both date to the late 1940s. The bag, inherited by the author, is valued at $95-115. The shoe heels feature the same carved Lucite as the lid of the bag, but are far less pricey in today's market, making them a good collectible at $25-55.

Left: Black and white is always right! The scallop top line of these pumps echoes the jaunty beret, circa 1955. *Courtesy of Lottie Ballou.* Value, shoes: $55-75.

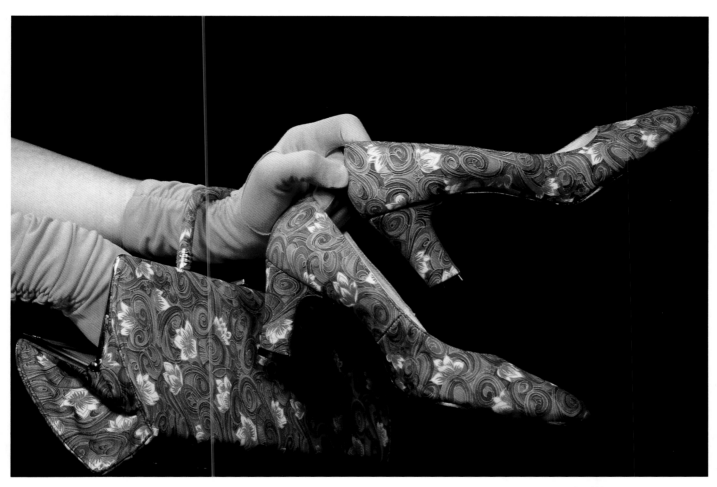

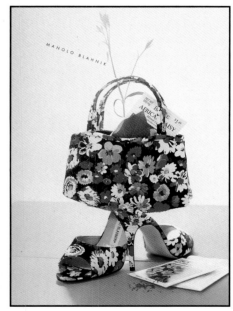

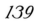

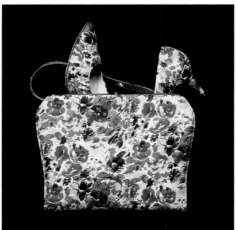

Above: An Op Art print lends drama to classic pumps and matching bag, circa 1965. *Courtesy of Lottie Ballou.* Value, the set: $45-65.

Right: Ready for a garden party, circa 1960, in a floral printed silk set. *Courtesy of Lottie Ballou.* Value: $35-55.

Who said sets are outré? In 1997, Manolo Blahnik brought back the garden party in matching mules and bag.

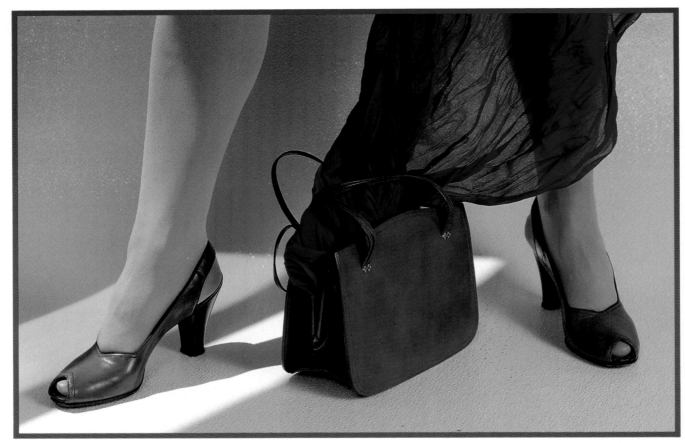

Kelly green kid slingbacks and boxy bag, a pulled-together springtime look for the mid-1950s. *Courtesy of Luxe.* Value: shoes, $35-55; bag, $45-65. *Courtesy of Luxe.*

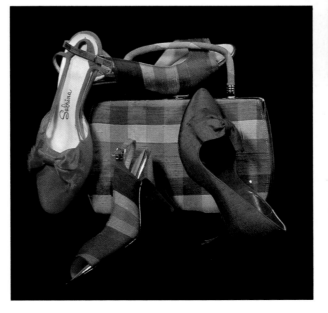

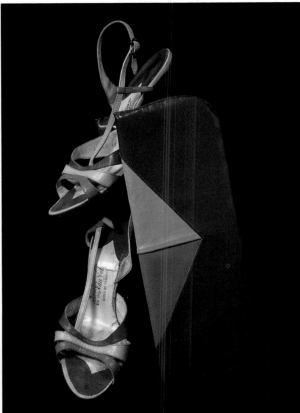

Above: Anchors aweigh, in a jaunty semaphore flat set from the late 1950s, from Lloyd Gotchy Shoes in Reno. *Courtesy of It's About Time.* Value, the set: $25-45.

Left: The blue pump shimmers with the unique iridescence of Thai silk, by Paradise Kittens, circa 1962. For special summer evenings, you can't beat the chic of the matched set in jewel-tone slubbed silk, from Barnetto's, circa 1967. The hot pink slingback with sassy fringed bow is by Sabrina, circa 1970. *Courtesy of The Blue Parrot, Barbara Grigg Vintage Fashions, and Lindy's Shoppe.* Value: blue, $35-55; pink, $15-25; set, $45-65.

SOUTH OF THE BORDER

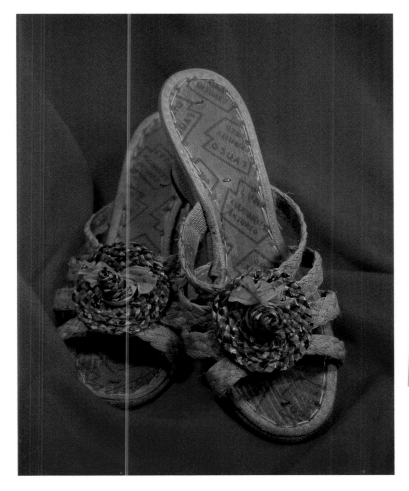

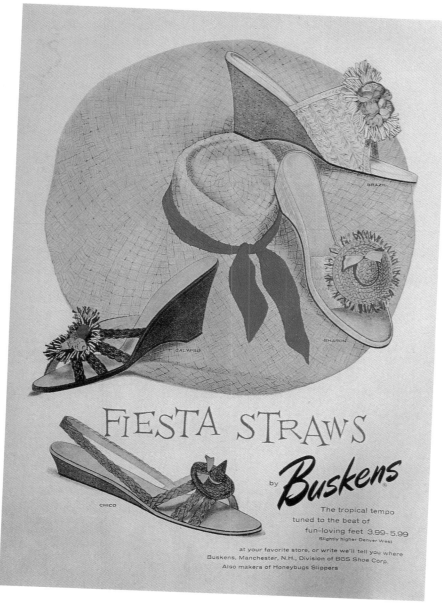

Do the Mexican Hat Dance in raffia wedgies! This pair is similar to Fiesta Straws, advertised by Buskens in the April 1958 issue of *Glamour* magazine: "The tropical tempo tuned to the beat of fun-loving feet (at) $3.99-$5.99. *Courtesy of It's About Time.* Value: $15-25.

South-of-the-Border still made a strong style statement in the 1950s, as shown in these dress pumps. The amusing drawstring bag makes a matched set in tooled cowhide. *Courtesy of It's About Time.* Value: shoes, $25-55; bag, $15-25.

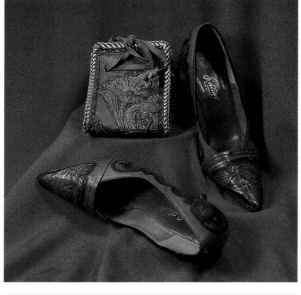

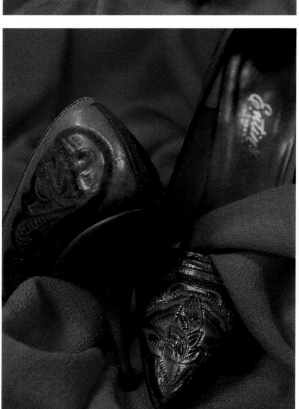

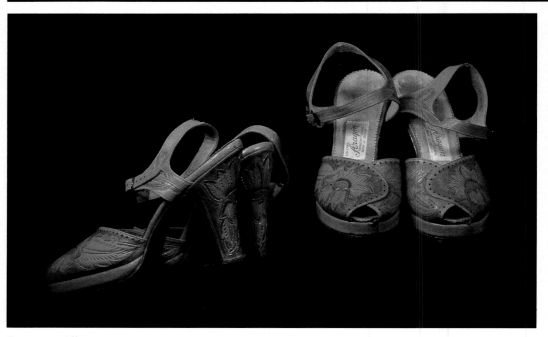

From two different collections, the popular hand-tooled cowhide slingback. Each pair is from the late 1940s, identical down to the Calzado, Aragon region of manufacture. *Collection of Laurie Gordon (left); collection of Sheryl Birkner (right).* Value: $25-55.

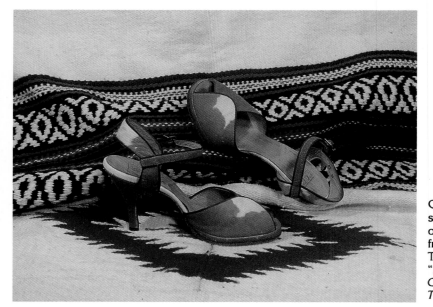

Cowhide never looked so good as on these open-toe slingbacks from the late 1940s. The label reads, "Fabrica de Calzad". *Courtesy of It's About Time.* Value: $25-55.

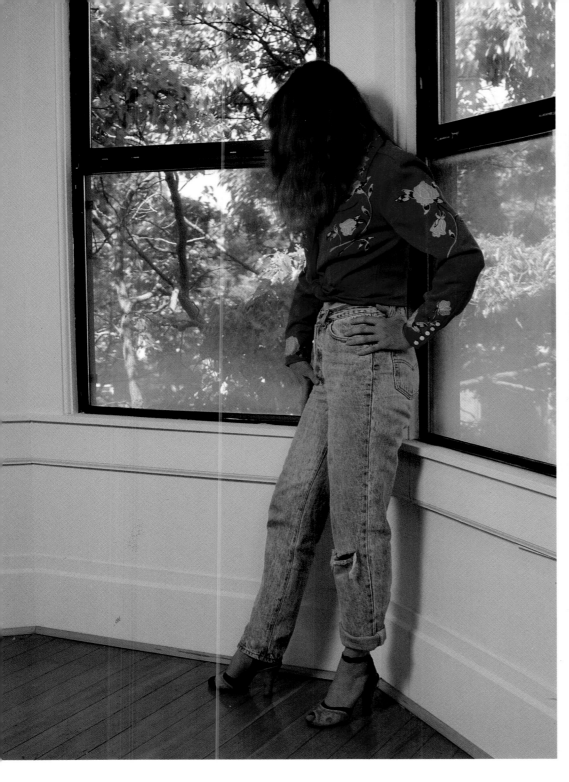

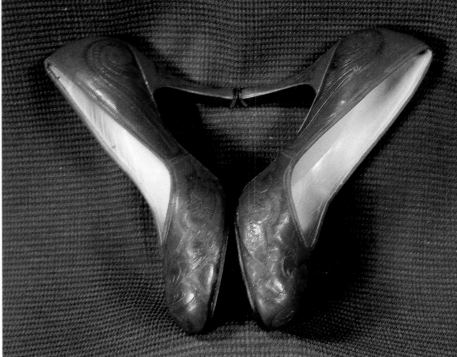

Above: Fiesta time! Who wouldn't feel festive in these red calfskin pumps, hand-tooled by an artisan for the Pipsa label. Made in Mexico, circa 1955. *Courtesy of Banbury Cross Antiques.* Value: $15-35.

Left: "I wear vintage shoes every day, they're better quality than modern. The old high heels are so well made, with inner arch supports and padding, I can walk or stand in them for hours." So says Pamela Joyce, and we believe her. She certainly looks at ease in a pair of hand-tooled leather and suede slingbacks, despite the soaring heels. Pamela also collects vintage cowgirl boots and is an accomplished rider. She was quick to explain that the rip in her jeans is not a fashion statement — but the result of skirmishing with a skittish horse, at her ranch in Northern California.

Chapter VIII

PARADE OF DECADES

Victorian and Edwardian
(1880–1910)

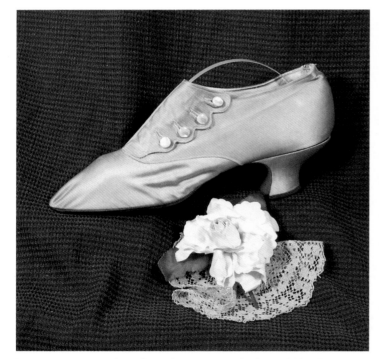

Ivory satin booties for a formal occasion in the late 1800s. They can be dated by the low-waisted Louis heel and by the fact that the mother-of-pearl buttons fasten on the outside of the ankle. Earlier booties would have had a flatter heel and would likely have laced up the inside ankle. *Collection of Carol Sidlow.* Value: Special.

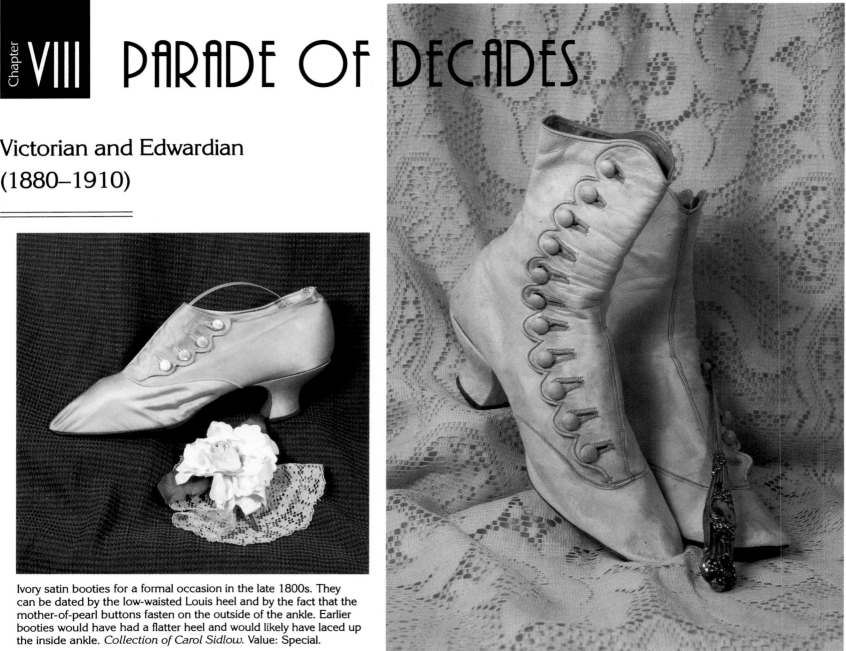

Purely beautiful shoes, fashioned from downy-white kid and fastened with high buttons in gleaming mother-of-pearl. It is tempting to speculate that they graced a bridal ensemble, but they might just as easily have been ordered for resort wear with a lingerie dress, circa 1890–1900. *Collection of Carol Sidlow.* Value: Special.

What could be more symbolic of Victorian womanhood than a high-button shoe? This endearing image has been cast in glass, sketched in artwork, and praised in song. It even formed the title of a smash Broadway musical!

For day, the Victorian woman usually wore high-button shoes of black or brown kid. In the summer, there was white or tan kidskin and canvas, or the combination of white canvas with black patent. For evening, the same seasonal colors prevailed, although a bronzed eggplant was also in vogue.

Collectors should also look for unique colors and fabrics in evening shoes of this era. Shoes certainly could be mass produced, but ladies of fashion would custom-order for a gala event. You may find high-button shoes in vivid shades of satin, and velvets or brocades. In the Gay Nineties, it was quite the fad for opera goers to wear ornately embroidered fabric booties, laced up the side of the ankle.

This palette would not alter much until a color explosion splashed across women's shoes after World War I. But when it came to color, what was absent earlier on in shoe color was made up for in the hosiery. Women had learned to flirt with the flare and dip of a hooped skirt, affording a glimpse of brilliantly patterned stockings.

Fancy hose were extremely popular with the Victorians, in patterns and colors that seem outrageous to the modern eye. There were bold tartans, vivid stripes, and jewel-toned argyles. The Edwardians favored stockings that were sprigged with floral embroidery or inset with lace. Beadwork, in clocks and garlands, was also popular. Stockings were knit in one piece from cotton lisle or silk then stitched to a separate foot of absorbent cotton. Although silk stockings were available in the 1880s, sheer silk would not make an appearance until the 1920s.

Hoops had been abandoned by the late 1880s, but the bustle took its place as an exaggeration of the female form. The silhouette was protruding in back, padded in front and wasp-waisted in the middle. Skirts

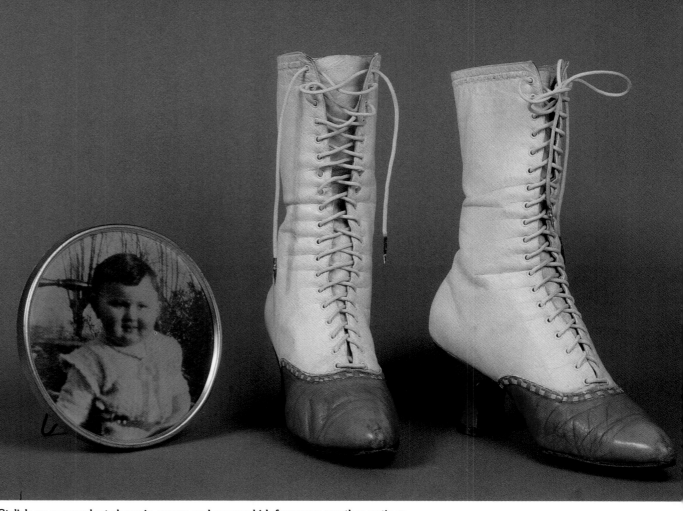

Stylish co-respondent shoes in cream and copper kid, for warm weather outings circa 1895–1905. *Courtesy of Rich Man, Poor Man.* Value: $155-175.

were draped and swagged, sweeping the floor by day, trailing a train by night. The high-buttoned shoe balanced this bulky silhouette, and its confinement of foot and ankle reflected the strict moral code of Queen Victoria's reign.

Morals and dress relaxed quite a bit during the brief years of the Belle Epoque following Queen Victoria's death in 1901 until her son King Edward's death in 1910. Edward well deserved his reputation as a racy *bon vivant* . His elegant queen, Alexandra, had the less dubious distinction of taste arbiter for women's fashion. She cut a fine figure in high-collared blouses and narrowly-cut skirts with demi-bustle. Under

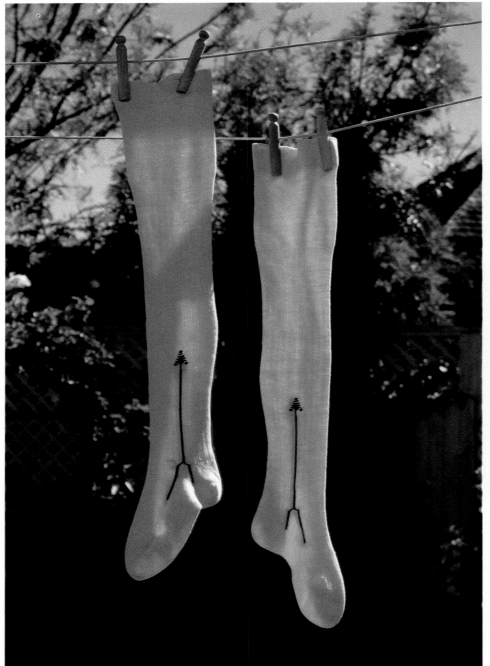

Woolen stockings air on the line, as they might have done 100 years ago. Note the decorative detail of black clocks, even though this was an "everyday" pair of hose. *Collection of Carol Sidlow.* Value: Special.

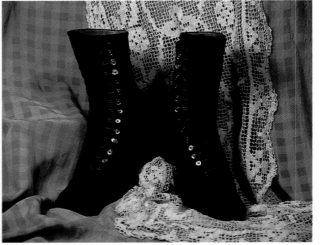

Mother-of-pearl buttons stream like ribbons down nut-brown velvet for a pair of dressy shoes from the Gay Nineties. *Collection of Carol Sidlow.* Value: Special.

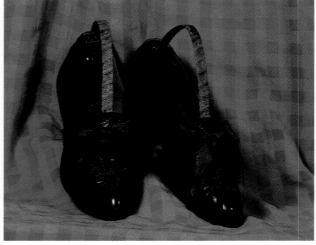

The ultimate shoe! Wine kid pumps, gussied up with a bronze beadwork cartouche and sassy grosgrain bow, circa 1915. If you are lucky enough to find such shoes, expect to pay upwards of $150, depending on condition. *Collection of Carol Sidlow.* Value: Special.

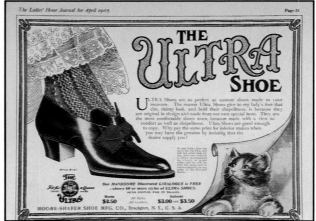

The ultimate shoe? In this ad from the April 1905 *Ladies' Home Journal.*, the Moore-Shafer Shoe Mfg. Co. boasted: "Ultra Shoes are as perfect as custom shoes made to your measure. The reason Ultra Shoes give to my lady's foot that chic, dainty look, and hold their shapeliness, is because they are original in design and made from our own special lasts." Boots or oxfords were priced at about $3.50.

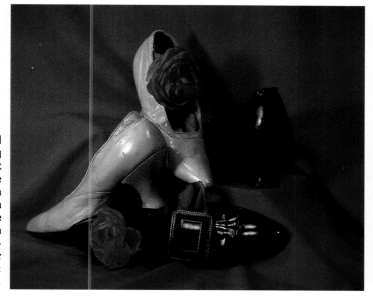

Two pair of kid pumps, reflecting the elegant simplicity of line that was favored in the Edwardian Era under the influence of Britain's Queen Alexandra. *Courtesy of Romantic Notions.* Value: $95-115.

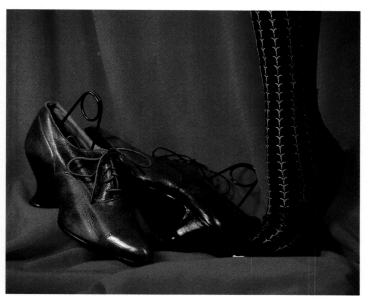

A sweet pair of oxfords, circa 1900–1910. Shoemakers were experimenting with exotic skins. Here, kid and reptile are combined in the colors of hot cocoa and fudge. They mix well with woolen stockings from the same era, in chocolate and cream. *Stockings courtesy of Lindy's Shoppe; shoes courtesy of The Blue Parrot.* Value: stockings, $25-35; shoes, $115-135.

her fashion tutelage, women began to explore the option of a low-buttoned shoe, and even a lace-up oxford for day; of a multi-bar shoe, or perhaps a pump, for night.

Queen Alexandra's jewels were extravagant, and the fabrics and laces used for her gowns were sumptuous. Following her example, women reveled in the sumptuous display of wealth during the Belle Epoque. This tendency was nowhere more manifest than in evening wear, with elaborate gowns further festooned with beading and plumage.

Like the gowns, the pumps of this era were also beaded to a fare-thee-well. Beadwork was in bronze, steel, or clear glass with the occasional glimmer of jet and marcasite. It usually decorated the vamp, although beading was also used to outline the throat of a shoe.

For dancing, pumps might be held on by silk or velvet ribbons, criss-crossed in the Grecian style, or closed by single- or multi-bar straps that buttoned across the instep. The latter style, the *barrette*, offered yet another surface area for beadwork.

High-button shoes were still worn during the Belle Epoque. For day, ladies favored the look of mock spats, with canvas for the boot part and leather for the shoe. Boots were also worn for evening, fashioned from glove-soft kid or satin, with a row of beaded *barrettes* parading up the shin.

The ubiquitous high-button shoe is still widely available to collectors in its various permutations of leather, canvas, and velvet. Likewise, oxfords and pumps, the latter with or without buckles in strass and filigree, are often available in new\old stock, or at least in mint condition. Beaded shoes and boots are more likely to be frayed, if only from repeated handling, but they still make a beautiful addition to any collection.

Don't expect to wear your acquisitions, though, even if you were so inclined. As would be expected, most shoes from the turn-of-the-century are small, the equivalent of a modern size 4 or 6. They are also extremely tight . Narrow feet were a sign of breeding and gentility. Both ladies and gentlemen suffered their feet to be laced into shoes or boots a full size too narrow. Even children wore tight, structured shoes almost from infancy to give proper support and to ensure that the foot did not widen unbecomingly.

After the anesthetic property of ether was discovered in the 1840s, *147* some ladies of fashion actually had their little toes surgically removed, for the vanity of a narrow foot. We are amazed today at the thought of such deformity. But is it all that far removed from the popular business of cosmetic liposuction?

Many collectors focus exclusively on Victorian childrens' shoes (think high-button booties with white china buttons). Victorian wedding slippers are another favorite, in ivory kid and satin. Often, in this sentimental era, they were deliberately left devoid of trim by the shoemaker since it was a common practice for the bride to secure her own, perhaps matched to her bouquet, or handed down from own mother's wedding.

Such chic shoes, to be worn with a walking suit circa 1900–1910. In drab olive kid with tan canvas uppers for comfort and a high-waisted heel for style. *Courtesy of Romantic Notions*. Value: $175-195.

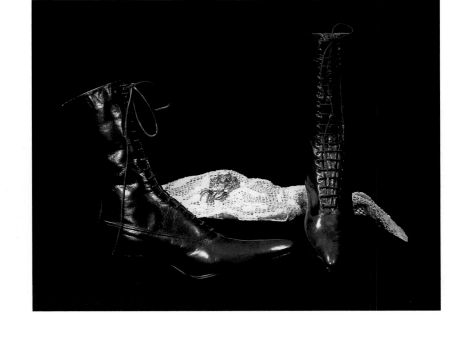

These old\new stock shoes are elegant at the burnished kid toe, but practical at the low, stacked wooden heel. They still bear a $62 price tag, quite dear in their day, which was circa 1900–1910. The original laces were leather cording, but one pair has been lost. *Courtesy of The Blue Parrot.* Value: $175-195.

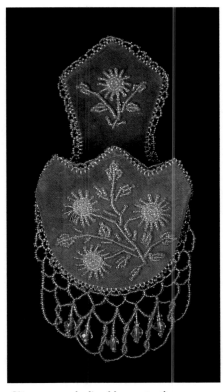

Slippers symbolized home to the Victorians, and were often shaped into decorative and useful items. This wallpocket was hand-beaded by a young lady for a church bazaar, circa 1910. It would have been hung near the bedpost, ready to receive a fob watch and chain at day's end.

Black wool stockings are sprigged with lilies-of-the-valley, the favorite flower of many a debutante in Old New York. The black single-bar shoes with twin buttons are set on waisted heels and feature an elongated toe, as was typical circa 1900–1910. *Courtesy of Romantic Notions.* Value: stockings, $35-45; shoes, $135-155.

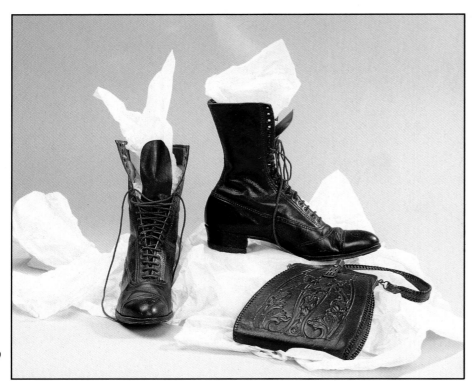

Sturdy walking shoes of the kind favored by active women at the turn-of-the-century. Shown with a sensible, embossed leather reticule. *Courtesy of Rich Man, Poor Man*. Value (shoes): $95-115.

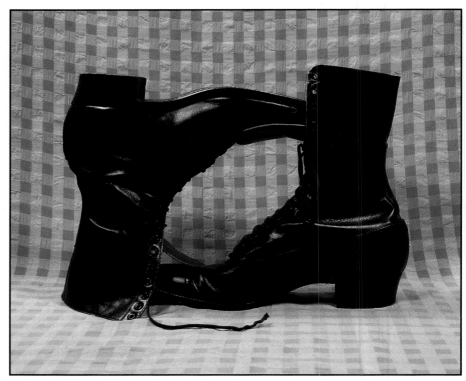

These boots were meant for walking! They are so simple and sensible, they may have been worn by a suffragette and could easily be worn by an active woman today. *Courtesy of Banbury Cross Antiques*. Value: $75-95.

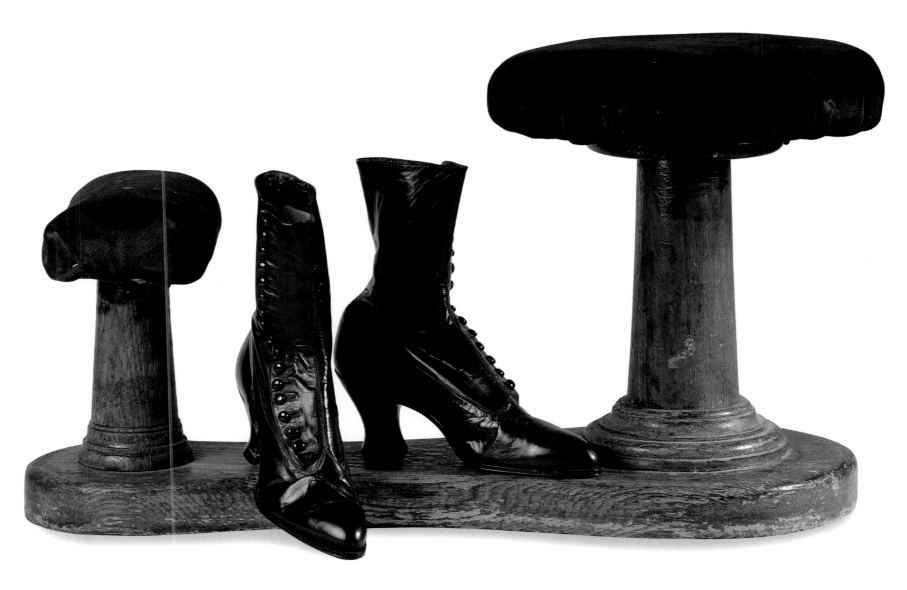

This remarkable footstool was used for the clientele of a Victorian shoe emporium. Presumably, *Madame* sat in a proper chair and the salesman shod her on the small pedestal in front of his padded stool. From the same era, glossy black high-button shoes in new\old stock, by Harry H. Gray's Son of Syracuse. *Courtesy of Lindy's Shoppe.* Value: stool, $175; shoes, $125-150.

The Teens (1911–1919)

The world was at war in 1914, a conflict that would last until the new decade dawned. The teens were years of strident social change, with well-bred women entering the work force for the first time in history. Dress reform followed by necessity: skirts were shortened, stays were loosened, and shoes were built for comfort.

At the same time, new methods of factory production had made it possible for women of average means to own more than one pair of *everyday* shoes. This placed a new emphasis on footwear as a fashion accessory. There were many experiments with materials and trim within the shape confines of a pointed toe, high-cut vamp, and waisted heel. The vamp was more rounded than in the Belle Epoque, and the toe less narrow and elongated. Altogether, it was an elegant and sensible silhouette.

A variety of materials were used and playfully mixed. Buckskin and antelope were shown with a canvas or gabardine top, buttoned to simulate spats. Leathers were reversed to form suede, which could be used in conjunction with a kid or patent finish. White kid and buckskin were standard for spectator sports, teamed with tan or black leather. These "spectators" were even worn by the sports participants, until canvas and rubber-soled shoes became available in the late teens.

For day, high-button shoes were still in style, especially during inclement weather.

For evening, there was the option of this boot or a court shoe, available in glacé kid and a full range of reptile skins (crocodile, snake, ostrich, even shark or shagreen). These leathers were dyed in elegant shades of dove, sand, olive, bronze, and eggplant. Of course, shoes could also be ordered in fabric, of the same satin or brocade used for a custom evening gown or dyed-to-match a walking suit.

The dress codes that dictated street wear relaxed quite a bit at home. By 1919, fashion magazines were showing hostess pajamas with pantaloon legs inspired by Paul Poiret's designs (in turn, based on costumes by Bakst for the Ballets Russe). These were meant to be worn with mules on little heels, perhaps with a satin rose at the toe; or flat slippers of brocade, or quilted satin.

152

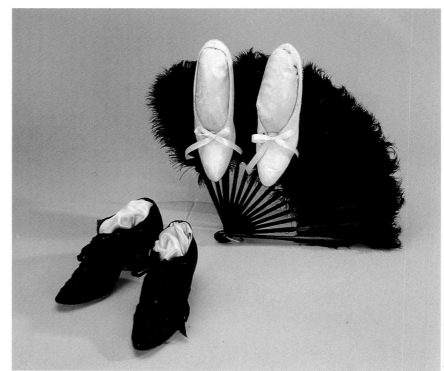

Two pair of silk shoes make a symphony in black and white, circa 1915. The top note of sequins and jet mark the oxfords for evening wear. *Courtesy of Rich Man, Poor Man.* Value: white, $55-75; black, $95-115.

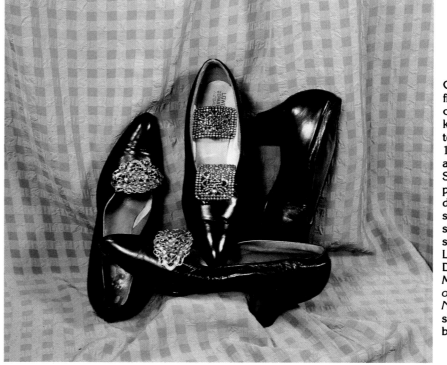

Cut steel and silver filigree buckles change plain black kid pumps from day to evening, circa 1915. These shoes are labeled "Lindke". Shown with a similar pair of pumps, dressed up with cut steel buckles. Those shoes are new\old stock from Lowenstein's Department Store in Michigan. *Courtesy of Romantic Notions.* Value: shoes, $75-95; buckles, $35-55.

For day or evening, pumps were shown with removable buckles in cut steel, silver filigree, strass, *diamonté*, and marcasite (which have collectible interest in their own right). These buckles grew more delicate in size, as the decade drew to a close.

The multi-bar boot was an alternative style for evening, each barrette fastened with the beauty mark of a jeweled button. Like all dressy shoes, these fanciful boots balanced on a high heel. The Cuban heel was advocated for wear at the balls and cotillions that formed many an evening's entertainment. But vanity prevailed and most dance shoes were slim and high.

Dancing was so popular that the evening hours weren't long enough and tea dancing became popular in mid-afternoon. Correct dress called for femininity and shoes were often tied around the ankle with satin ribbon. In kid or satin, these shoes were usually dyed-to-match the romantic sherbet colors of a full-skirted *robe de style*.

By the mid-teens, when skirts no longer grazed the floor, fashion's eye was on the stocking—cotton lisle for day with embroidered flowers; silk for evening with lace inserts or beadwork clocks. Sheer silk stockings were showcased by the editors of *Vogue* in 1911. For the daring, ribboned garters were worn just beneath the knee, intentionally visible with every movement of the skirt.

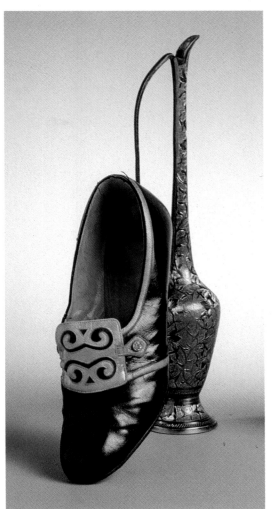

Left: Gold kid forms a faux filigree buckle on black kid court shoes, circa 1915–1920. *Courtesy of Past Perfect.* Value: $95-115.

Below: Black suede with a unique double-bar closure, low-heeled pumps for city streets circa 1915–1920. *Courtesy of Past Perfect.* Value: $75-95.

153

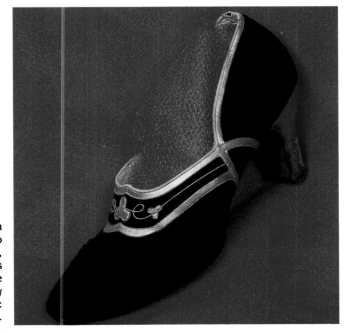

A lovely slipper in shattered black silk. So correct for the casino, with Lady Luck's insignia wrapping the vamp in gold. *Courtesy of Lottie Ballou.* Value: Special.

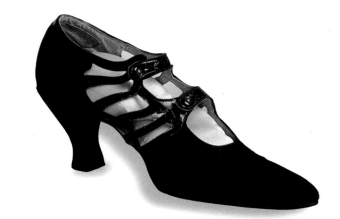

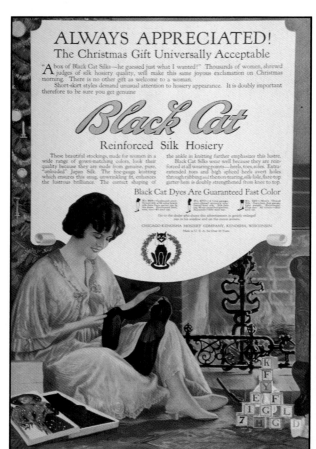

"A box of Black Cat Silks—he guessed just what I wanted!" So said this miss on Christmas morning, 1916. This brand of hose featured a "non-tearing, silk-lisle, flare-top garter-hem . . . doubly strengthened from knee to top."

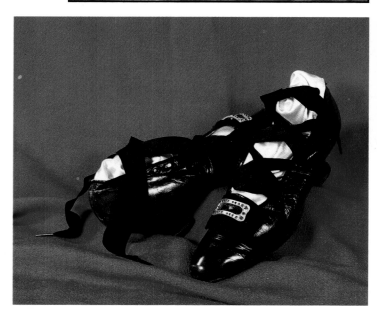

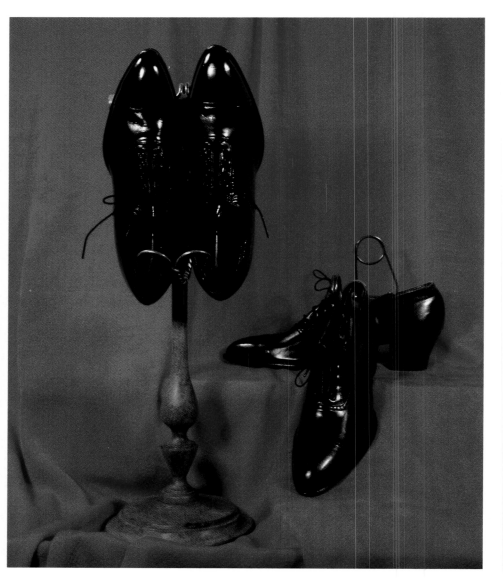

Above: Shoebox fresh, black and brown leather oxfords, warehoused since the mid-teens by a defunct department store in Milwaukee. The wooden shoetrees are old store display items of the same era. *Collection of Romantic Notions.* Value: shoes, $95-115; shoetrees, $35-55.

Left: According to fashion periodicals in the early teens, the "smart set" wore a photo of their lovers at the toe of their shoes, fixed by criss-crossing velvet ribbons. The style shown here would have been ideal for such a purpose. (Note: the authentic laces are of silk jersey.) *Courtesy Lottie Ballou.* Value: Special.

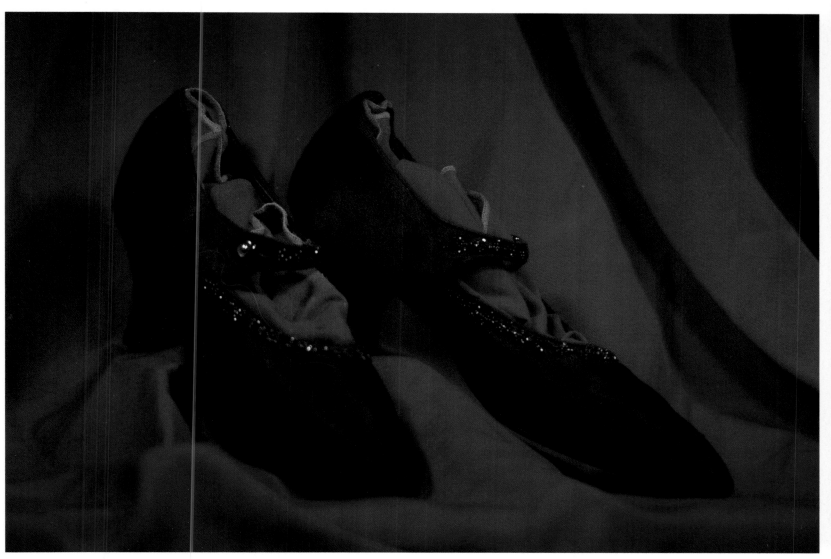

Above: Sapphire blue beads brighten a pair of black satin single-bar evening pumps, circa 1910–1915. *Courtesy of The Blue Parrot.* Value: $165-185.

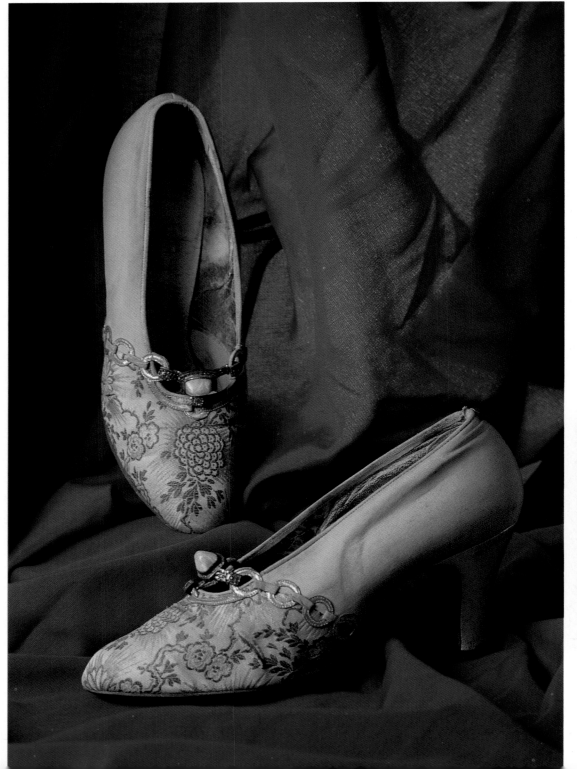

The Jazz Age
(1920-1929)

The war was over, and Americans who had fought overseas came home with expanded views about the arts and culture. The general mood was lighter, more experimental, than in the preceding two decades and this emancipated attitude was reflected in women's clothing.

Dresses pared down to the simple lines of a chemise, with hem lines just below the knees. The flirty flapper would roll her stockings down and rouge her knees for a naughty schoolgirl effect.

Stockings might be black cotton, silk, or lace. In the early '20s, black was still appropriate for day, along with flesh tones. In 1925, American factories cranked out some 12,300,000 dozen pairs of stockings—a dramatic increase of almost one-hundred percent over 1919. Production techniques also improved. Earlier stockings had been knit like a tube. They were seamless, but baggy at the knees and ankles. The new stock-

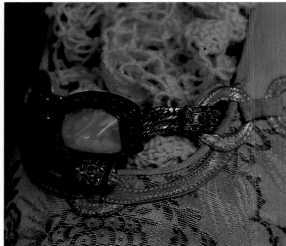

According to the former owner, these fabulous evening pumps were originally made for a friend of silent movie star Mary Pickford in the early 1920s. They're ready to vie with any screen legend for drama, in satin and silk brocade with a jewel-encrusted swoop of swashbuckle. *Courtesy of Lindy's Shoppe.* Value: Special.

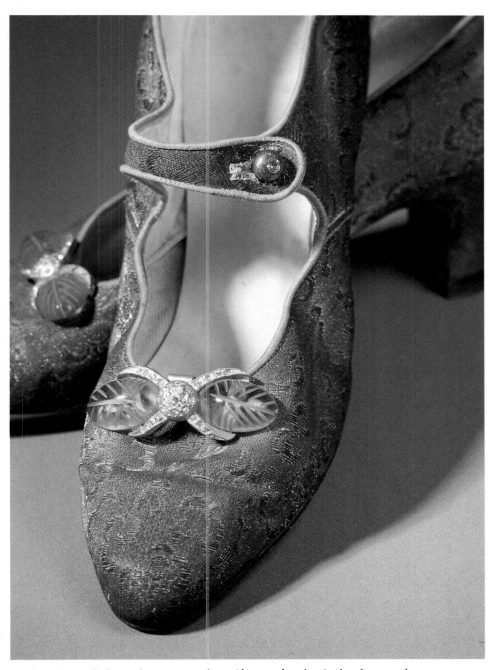

ings were in two shaped pieces with a seam down the back. More expensive to make, but infinitely more desirable to wear.

In this country, hose could not be sheer enough for both day and evening. The French continued to favor clocks, lace, and *millefiori* patterning. For sports, fashion periodicals showed argyle wool hose with low-heeled oxfords and spectators.

The shift in dress proportions caused great interest in pretty and unusual shoes. For the first time, shoe uppers were cut low and featured cut-outs at vamp and sides. Quite a departure from the days when a glimpse of stocking was simply shocking!

Throughout the decade, there were many experiments with hem lines and silhouettes, including shifts in shoe styles. Shoes featured high tongues in 1922, cutaways in 1923, T-straps and crossover straps in 1924. The most common shoe of the era was a single-bar pump, with pointed toe and high, waisted heel. Common, yes; ordinary, never.

This decade produced some of the most exciting shoes of all time. There was great innovation in the use of bright fabrics, and brilliantly-dyed leather. At night, silver and gold came out to play in glacé kid, brocade, and satin. Luxurys

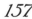

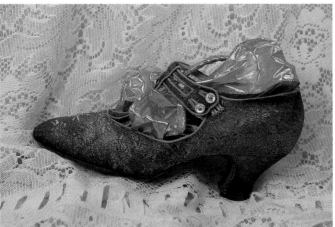

Above: A demure opera pump in dove-gray cloth, with a beaded bow as its only ornament. Simple and charming, by Fenton Footwear for Saks Fifth Avenue, circa 1925. *Courtesy of Barbara Grigg Vintage Fashions.* Value: $55-75.

157

Luminous silk brocade pumps, aglow with carved amber in the shape and color of cats' eyes. Given the opulence of these Bakelite and diamontè clips, no doubt the buttons were treated to jeweled covers, which would have been sold separately like the clips. These shoes are by an unknown designer of the mid-20s. *Courtesy of Vintage Silhouettes.* Value: $95-115.

Single-bar shoes with twin mother-of-pearl buttons in a sophisticated shade of pewter. The metallic brocade was most likely imported from France for use by an unknown shoe designer, circa 1925. *Collection of Richard and Sylvia Unger.* Value: Special.

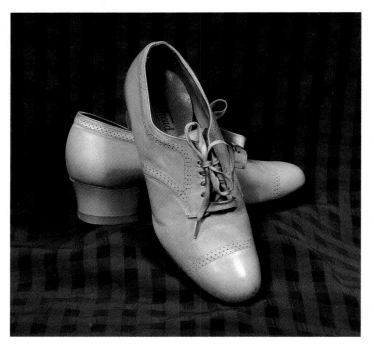

materials were layered to fantastic effect. Rich brocade was over-stitched with metallic thread; satin and silk was hand-gilded, embroidered, and beaded; velvet was cut like a jacquard, or quilted with gold braid. These jewel-tones were shown with a full range of jeweled trim.

Flappers who danced the Charleston needed some assurance that their shoes would not fly off with every high-stepping kick. Thus a new style of dance shoe was born. The heel was lowered, the toe was closed, and the vamp was securely strapped. For glamour, this shoe depended on material and trim.

Buckles gleamed with rhinestones and even semi-precious stones. Fabulous heels were the height of fashion, crafted with a jeweler's skill. Bakelite heels might be carved or studded with rhinestones. Leather heels might be quilted or overlaid with lace. Women even walked, carefully, on heels made entirely of Wedgwood and Jasperware.

Plain court shoes could be dressed-up with removable buckles. These were initially quite bold, although they grew discreet by the late '20s. Pearls and *diamonté* were correct for evening, silver and mother-of-pearl for day. Bronze appeared in 1922, and sequins in 1924. Shoemakers also used engine-turned metals, enamel, and *guilloche*. By 1926, shoes were also trimmed

Above: Trim white kid oxfords with stacked wooden heel, Cuban style. A serviceable shoe, circa 1929. *Author's collection.* Value: $45-65.

Left: Oxfords are enduring, witness these classics from the late 1920s in basic black and white kid. Value: $55-65. *Courtesy of Rich Man, Poor Man.*

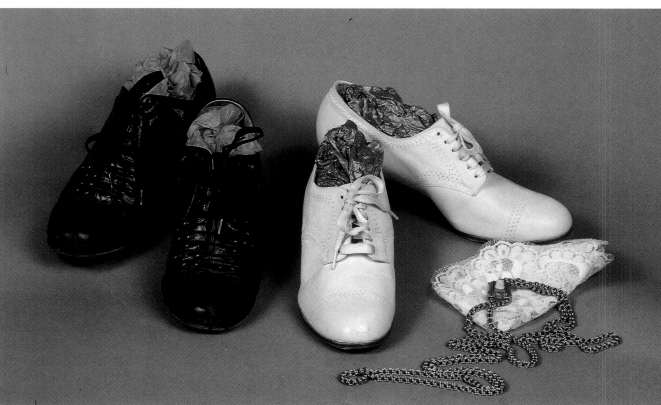

with large semi-precious stones, colored rhinestones, faceted onyx, and cut crystal.

Throughout the '20s, women used tiny button covers to decorate the plain fastening of a single-bar strap. These were often engraved metal or marcasite, styled in the geometric art deco manner.

Shoe designers experimented with a mix of leather with fabric and leather treated like fabric. The refinement of aniline dyes meant that leather could be treated to infinite varieties of color. Early in the decade, vivid hues were in vogue. Shoes might be cherry red, canary yellow, jade green, royal blue, or deep plum. These colors might be used to punctuate white or black, for a strong contrast at vamp or heel, or in a duotone palette of bright brown and yellow, red and blue, green and plum.

The same care went into low-heeled mules for little evenings at home. Fur cuffs or silk cockades might be added to the vamp of a flat-heeled velvet slipper.

By the mid-1920s, the novelty of color had worn off. Shoes were shown in subtle shades of gray, brown, and bone. White buckskin was popular, often perforated or topstitched for a sporty look; it was also teamed with brown or navy for spectators. Reptile was still popular, for the allover shoe or as inserts at the tongue or T-strap.

Leather was treated to a myriad of finishing processes, some quite new. For years, shoes were available in patent, suede, or polished kid. Now they could also be made in glacé or argenté, kid, or snakeskin. Perugia had leather hand-painted with flowers and geometric forms. Hellstern developed a pyrographic technique for embossing and over-dying leather.

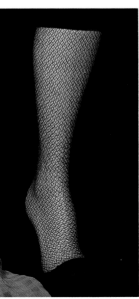

Right: Silk netting was fashionable in the teens as a dressier alternative to wool, like the russet stocking shown. Black silk stockings had been available since the teens, but the sheer silks were to come later. *Courtesy of Lindy's Shoppe.* Value: $25-45.

Far right: These fawn suede pumps are classics, from their perforated toes to the stacked wooden heels. Made for town or country circa 1929, and just as stylish a half-century later. By Rose Marie, as shown on the original, and charmingly illustrated, shoebox. *Courtesy of Sylvia and Richard Unger.* Value: Special.

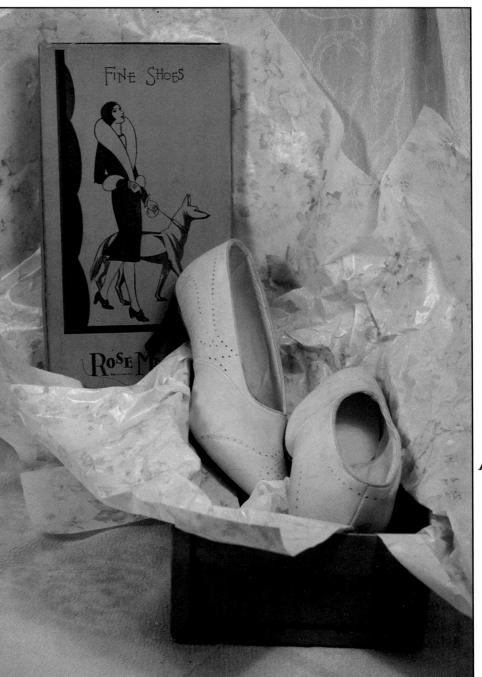

Low-button shoes such as these co-respondents would have been worn with country tweeds in the late teens or early 1920s. (If the heels were waisted, instead of straight, they would be even earlier.) *Courtesy of Lindy's Shoppe.* Value: $75-95.

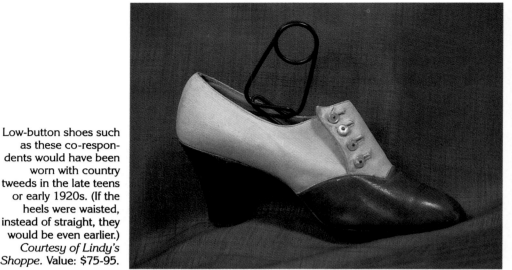

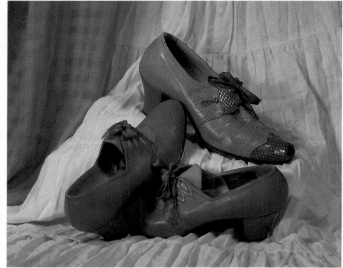

Look-alike oxfords in tan kid and snake-skin from the mid-1920s. The cap-toe style is by Dickerson, the other is by Cantilever Shoes. Value: Special. *Collection of Sheryl Birkner.*

Well-worn spectators in navy kid and ivory mesh by Enna Jetticks, a label long associated with comfortable footwear. The lace-up vamp was deliberately made sans tongue to provide an amusing glimpse of stockings in the late 1920s. *Collection of Sylvia and Richard Unger.* Value: Special.

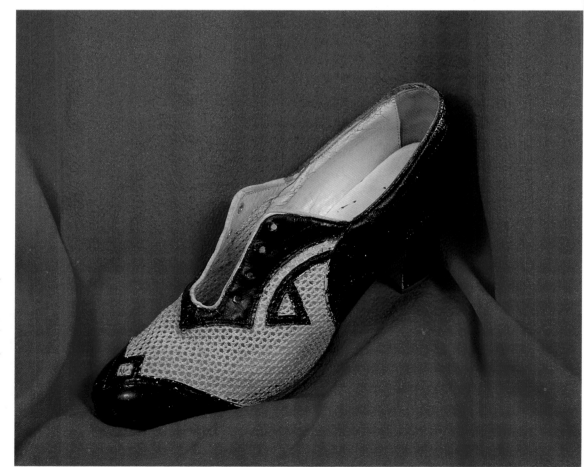

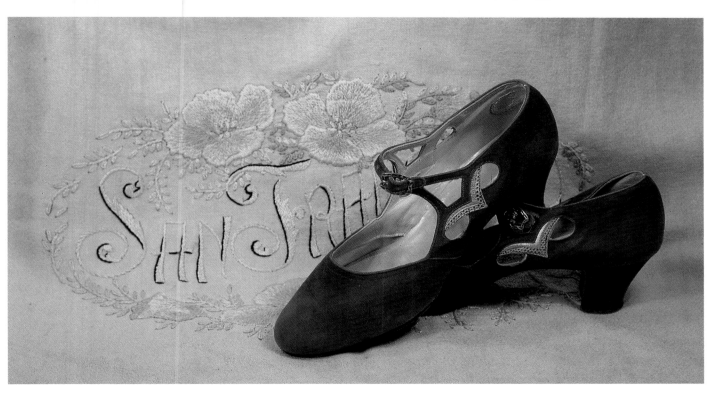

From a G. H. Baker shoe store in San Francisco, circa 1922: brown suede single-bar pumps with lizard insets for interest. *Collection of Sylvia and Richard Unger.* Value: Special.

The elongated toe and high Louis heel of the late teens continued into the early 1920s, as featured in this ad by Queen Quality in the May 1921 issue of *Pictorial Review*. The sales pitch is timeless, if a bit high-flown: "Look at your hand in a well-cut glove—then at your feet in Queen Quality shoes—and you will realize an equal perfection in fit and beauty."

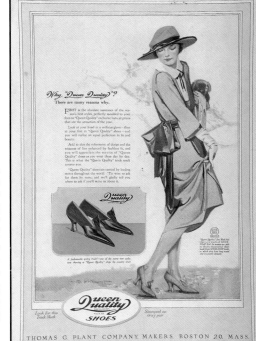

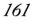

Basic black sateen pumps with brilliant buckles by Lubin's of Detroit, circa 1925–1930. *Collection of Richard and Sylvia Unger.* Value: Special.

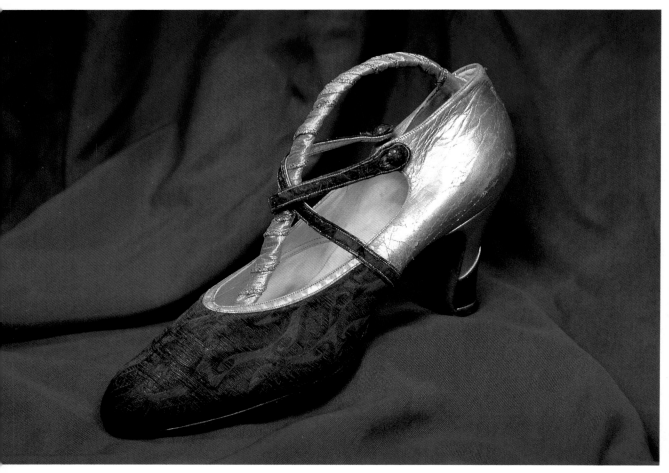

Like Lanvin's trademark perfume bottle, these shoes are redolent of an *Evening in Paris*. In sapphire-blue brocade and silver kid, by Sandalari circa 1925. These shoes were sold from a Parisian *boitier* at 364 Rue St. Honore. *Collection of Richard and Sylvia Unger.* Value: Special.

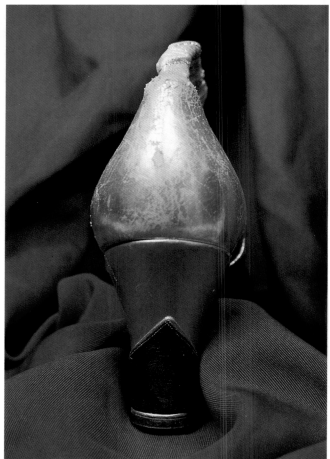

Modern Times (1930–1939)

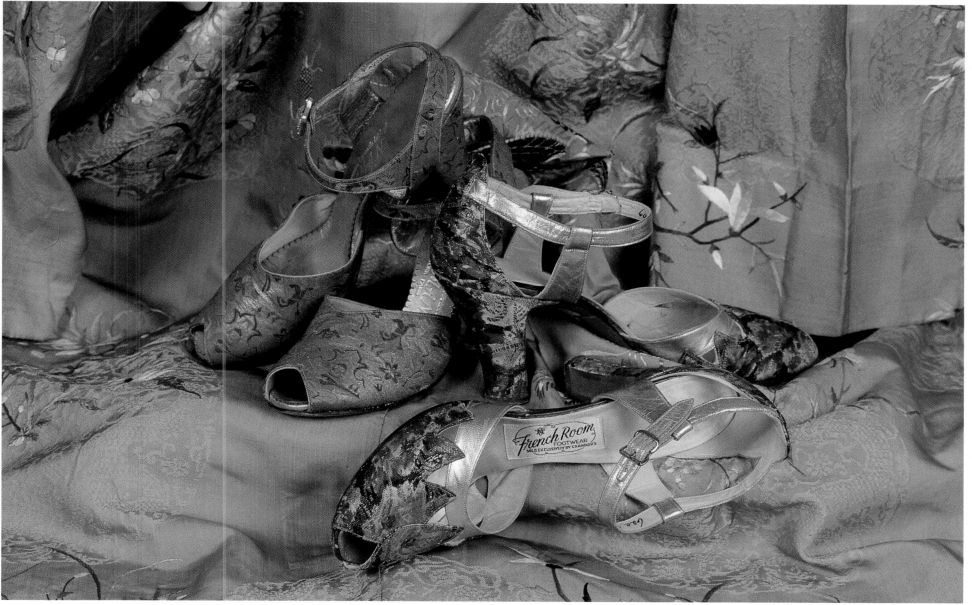

Rich and exotic brocades conjure up images of Arabia. These dance shoes have a touch of the harem Hollywood-style, from the mid-1930s. The foreground pair are from The French Room at Chandler's; in the background are Paris imports by Delman. *Courtesy of Lottie Ballou.* Value: $25-55 and $75-95, respectively.

The Great Depression became noticeable almost immediately in the garment industry.

With less money to spend, the 1930s woman shied from imported fabrics and luxury trim, relying instead on the timeless natural waistline with the fluidity of a bias-cut. Perhaps to compensate for this simplicity of line in her dress, her shoes were dazzling in their variety and sophistication.

In general, the silhouette was less extreme than in the '20s. Toes were rounded; heels were slightly curved, and lowered. Shoes were also cut higher in the vamp, creating the beloved "chubby" look of 1930s footwear. But the 1930s woman could choose from high, low, or no heel; décolleté or high-tongued vamp; T-strap or ankle strap; sling-back or backless—all in a bewildering array of leathers, fabrics, and trim.

When the event was after-five, ladies changed into cutaway pumps or sling-back sandals in brilliant silks and satins. The same style segued into formal wear with the embellishment of metallic kid and rhinestones. Jeweled buckles were still shown, along with jewel-studded Bakelite heels. High heels remained as essential to a woman's allure as her lipstick and perfume.

In the early '30s, designers continued to draw inspiration from art deco. For example, pumps might feature the swoop of an asymmetric strap across each instep. Sandals, flat or heeled, were formed from multiple straps that zigzagged up the vamp. By the late '30s, the surrealist movement in art was increasingly evident. Raft-soled sandals were shown by Schiaparelli, and mock sweater ankle boots were knit by Perugia.

For the first time, casual wear was an acceptable mode of dress. It's almost as if the rules of fashion decorum relaxed, when the economy crashed. Women began wearing slacks with loafers and flat sandals. It was an ideal way to dress for those who could no longer afford a maid to clean, cook, and run errands. The look was fresh, clean, and all-American.

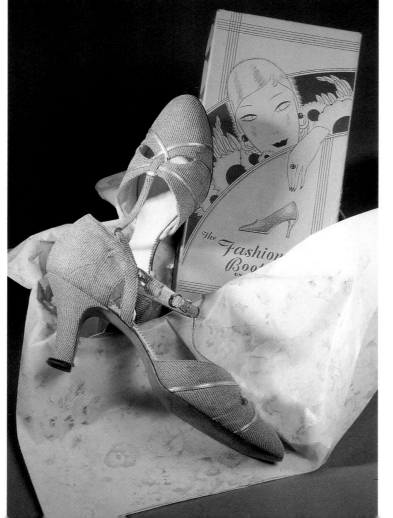

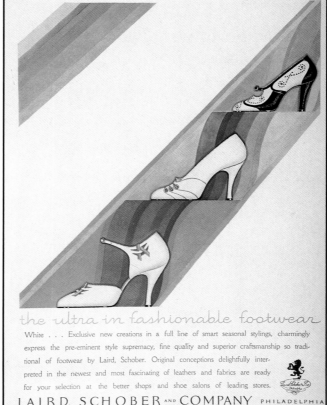

Left: For the spring of 1932, a trio of light and bright shoes from Laird, Schober & Co.

Far left: Ladylike textured linen T-straps, with the surprise of silver kid, from The French Room at Chandler's circa 1920–25. Shown with a shoebox of the same era from The Fashion Bootery. *Collection of Sheryl Birkner.* Value: Special.

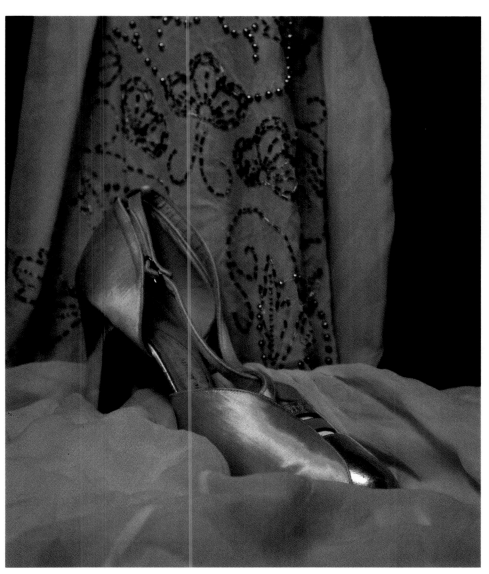

Drink a toast from champagne satin shoes, lit up with silver kid at toe and heel. Bearing The White House label, these shoes are from the late 1920s or early 1930s. *Courtesy of Barbara Grigg Vintage Fashion.* Value: $75-95.

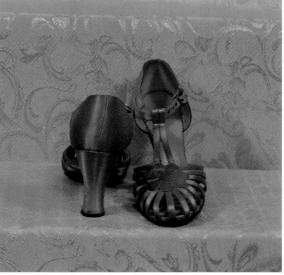

Pale blue satin T-strap dance pumps by Paris Stuart, circa 1930–1935. *Courtesy of Banbury Cross Antiques.* Value: $35-55.

The casual trend was reinforced by a growing national interest in sports and outdoor activities. A new sportswear industry began showing specialty shoes for tennis, skiing, and golfing. Most women owned at least one pair of clogs or moccasins for a trip to the mountains, along with canvas espadrilles for the beach and flat sandals for the country.

This is not to say that the public accepted sloppiness of attire. Fashion magazines emphasized the importance of dressing "correctly" for the occasion. For business in town, this meant closed-toe leather pumps, sturdy of heel and high of vamp. For sports it was suede ghillies or mesh-and-leather oxfords. For summer, after Labor Day, there were bright sandals and white oxfords with mesh inserts. For fall, after Memorial Day, the palette changed to black, brown, and navy pumps and sling-backs. Black linen was always in season for day, as was gold or silver kid for evening.

By 1932, new technologies had made sheer silk hose widely available. This ushered in a fad for peep-toe shoes, a fad that would last two decades. The sling-back was another favorite. These two were often combined to expose milady's foot more than ever before, not just in the evening sandal but also in the street pump.

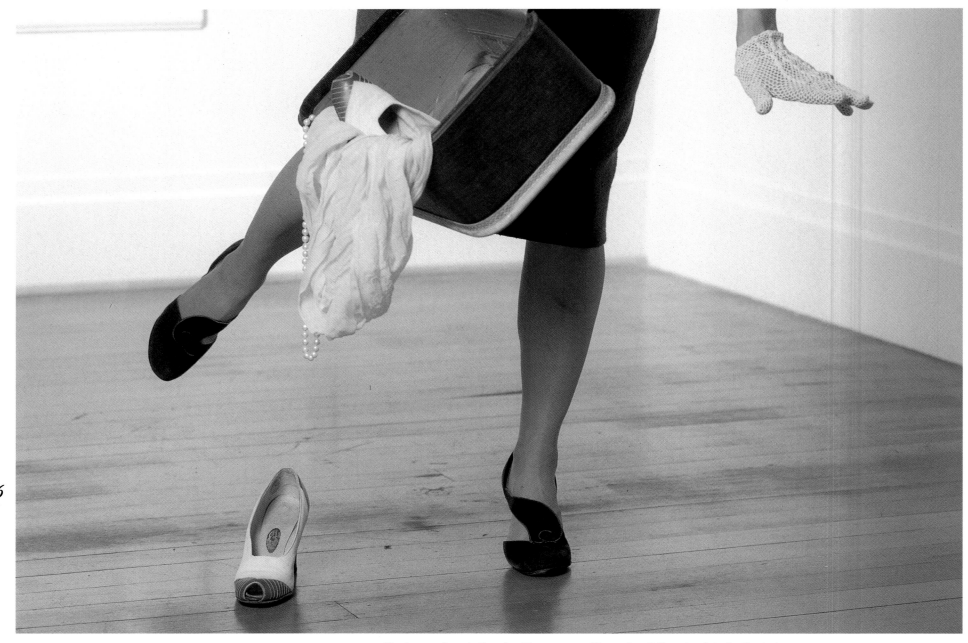

Pardon me boy, is that the Chattanooga Choo-choo? Running late for the train, in swoopy green suede by Smartest Collegiene. Dropping from the train case: spectator slingbacks by Paradise Shoes. Value: $55-75 and $35-55 respectively. *Suede shoes courtesy of Luxe; spectators courtesy of Lindy's Shoppe.*

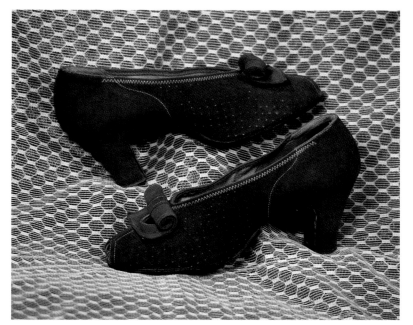

Chubbies in forest green suede with peep toe and perforations, from the early 1930s. *Courtesy of Time After Time*. Value: $45-65.

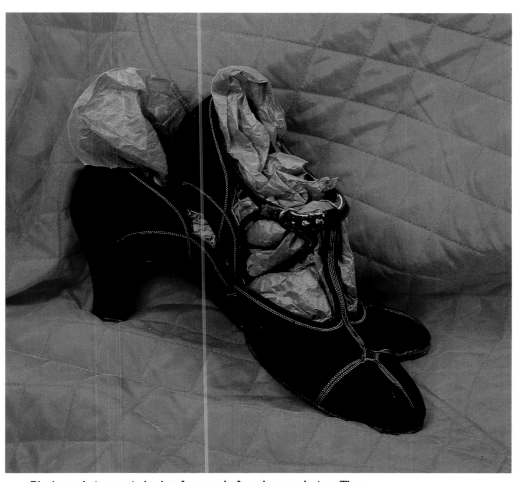

Black suede is topstitched to form a shaft and arrow design. These shoes were touted as exclusive to H. C. Capwell's department store, circa 1930. *Collection of Sylvia and Richard Unger*. Value: Special.

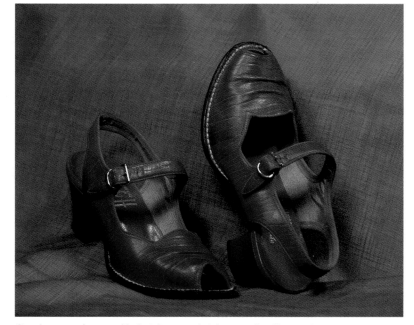

Cranberry red crocodile brightens a brisk pair of walkers, circa 1930–1935. *Collection of Sheryl Birkner*. Value: Special.

Humming Bird Hose advertised its wares in 1932 with great attention to detail. There was "the quality of the silk, the twist of the thread, the closeness of texture, the trimness of finish, inside and outside." The company promoted nine styles, including "a very simple mesh for formal wear." With this kind of variety, silk stockings must have been purchased by many, despite the relatively dear price of $1-1.95 a pair.

In February 1938, *Vogue* ran its annual *Americana* issue with an article on "America—Feet First." The editors culled statistics from some obscure government survey, to create this arresting image of the consumer as patriot:

"The stirring words 'Thank God, America is an extravagant nation' have been attributed variously to several gentlemen—(who love) the invariably silk-clad legs, the unfailingly pretty shoes of our army of American women.

"For compared with other nations we are, obviously, extravagant about our shoes and stockings. We buy silk stockings for beauty only; we don't even hope that they will wear very long. Nowhere else in the world are silk stockings worn constantly as they are here. Nowhere else is every pair of female legs flattered by silk stockings every day.

"Last year, forty million women, between them, bought one hundred and eighty million pairs of shoes—roughly speaking, four and one-half pairs apiece. [To be] compared with the British who buy not quite two pairs each year; with the French, who average a pair and a half; with the Germans, who buy one and one-tenth pairs . . ."

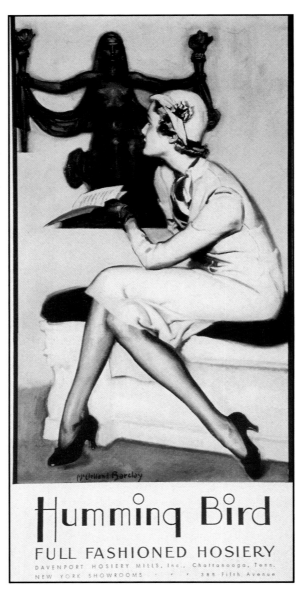

Humming Bird
FULL FASHIONED HOSIERY
DAVENPORT HOSIERY MILLS, Inc., Chattanooga, Tenn.
NEW YORK SHOWROOMS · · · 385 Fifth Avenue

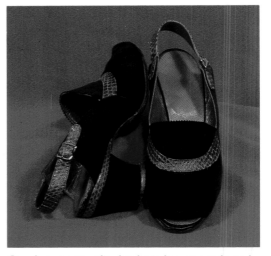

Comfy open-toe slingbacks in brown suede and snakeskin, set on Cuban heels. These walking shoes are from the mid- to late 1930s. *Courtesy of Banbury Cross Antiques.* Value: $25-35.

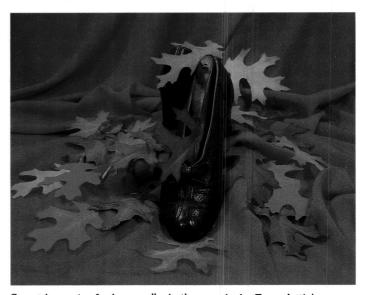

Sweet brownies for long walks in the woods, by Enna Jettick circa 1935. *Courtesy of It's About Time.* Value: $25-35.

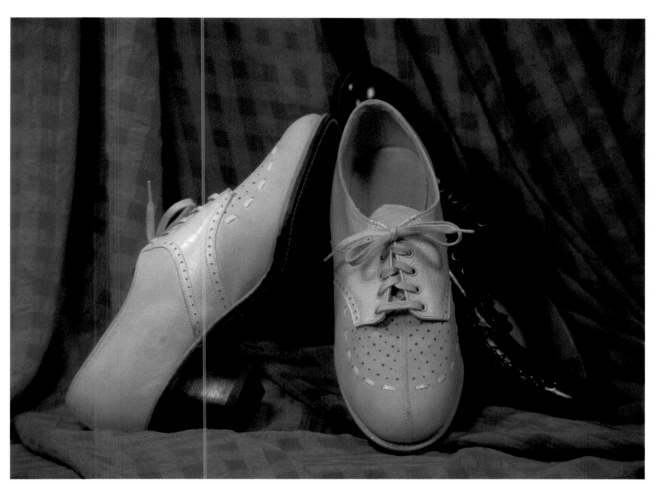

Not quite a spectator, almost a saddle shoe—in creamy croc and *café au lait* kid. Note the perforated toe, bold topstitching, and stacked wood heel on this new\old stock shoe. By Buck Hecht Brogue, circa 1935. *Courtesy of The Blue Parrot.* Value: $55-75.

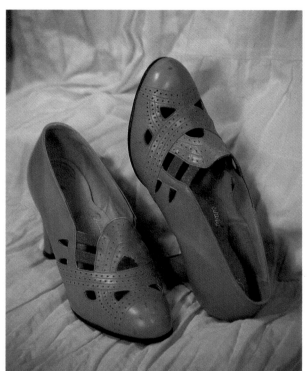

From Boulevard Styles, a pair of taupe pumps for boulevard strolls circa 1930. Elastic inserts stretched with the wearer's stride; perforated leather gave good air circulation. *Courtesy of Vintage Silhouettes.* Value: $45-65.

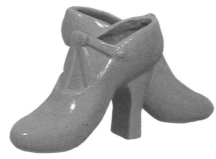

Twin T-straps in high-glaze lemon yellow china, amusing for display on a whatnot, circa 1935. *Courtesy of Rich Man, Poor Man.* Value: $25.

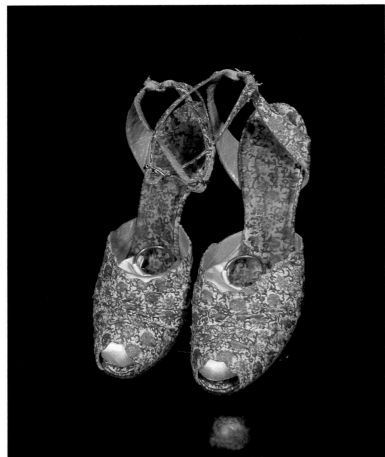

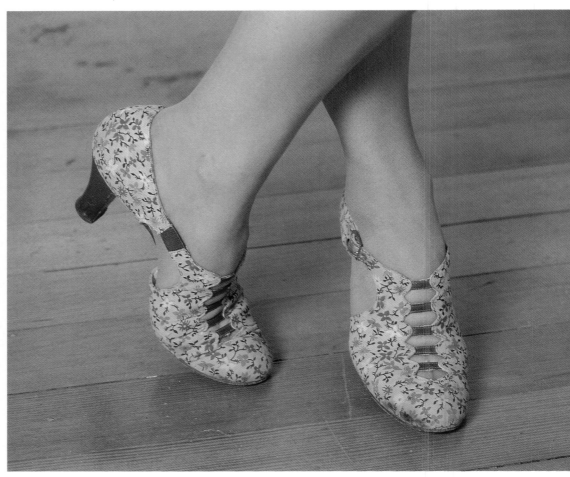

Pretty and practical, *millefleur* fabric ankle strap shoes from the mid-1930s. *Collection of Laurie Gordon.* Value: Special.

Cheery yellow calico goes from country to city when fashioned into smart high-vamp pumps like these. The label is Zesman's, the era is late 1930s. *Courtesy of Past Perfect.* Value: $65-75.

Right: I. Miller advertised *COLOR* in Spring 1937. Note the charming tradition of naming each style (which seems to have followed in the steps of *haute couture* collections). The Nasturtium Yellow shoe is named Zenophobia, the Canterbury Blue is Tallulah, the Dahlia Red is Butterfly. The multi-color shoes are (left to right) Swing, Cyprus, and Guatemala.

Below: Just like Ginger Rogers, these red suede sandals are feisty, flirty, and ready to dance all night. By Ansonia Deluxe, circa 1935. *Courtesy of Lottie Ballou.* Value: $35-55.

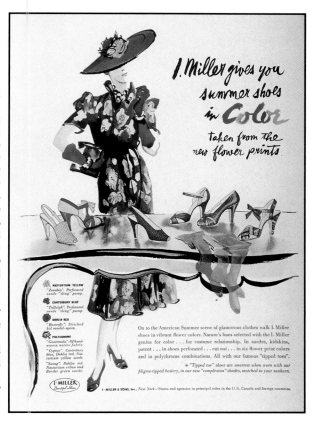

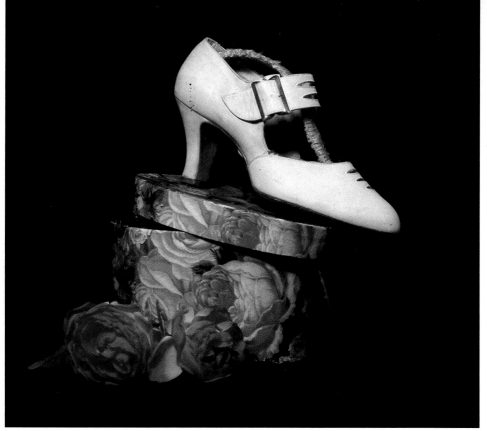

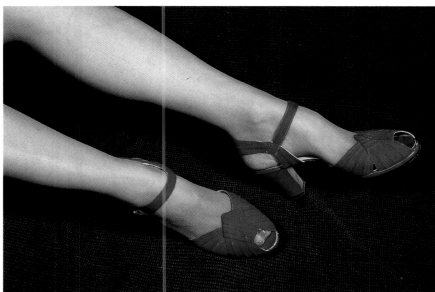

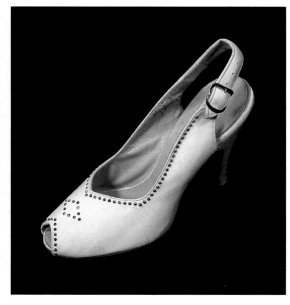

Above: White suede pumps buckled by a bold single bar are *moderne* . This classic style would have been just right for summer frocks in the early 1930s. *Courtesy of Vintage Silhouettes.* Value: $35-55.

Left: Multicolored metal beads spill across white suede, an amusing contrast for springtime in the late 1930s. A few years later and these slingbacks would have had platform soles. Crafted by Frank More of San Francisco, in a diminutive size 4. *Author's collection.* Value: $55-75.

Many women seek out vintage shoes to accessorize their clothing. Such is the case for Sheryl Birkner, who models for special fashion events by the Art Deco Society of San Francisco. She is shown here in a bias-cut dress and green cobra slingbacks by Troylings, from her own collection. "I started buying vintage shoes in the late 1960s, when I was a student in college. Perpetually broke, I couldn't afford the newly hip platforms in the department stores. Much to my surprise, I found out that I could get even funkier 1940s platforms for about 50 cents at the Goodwill." Ah, those were the days.

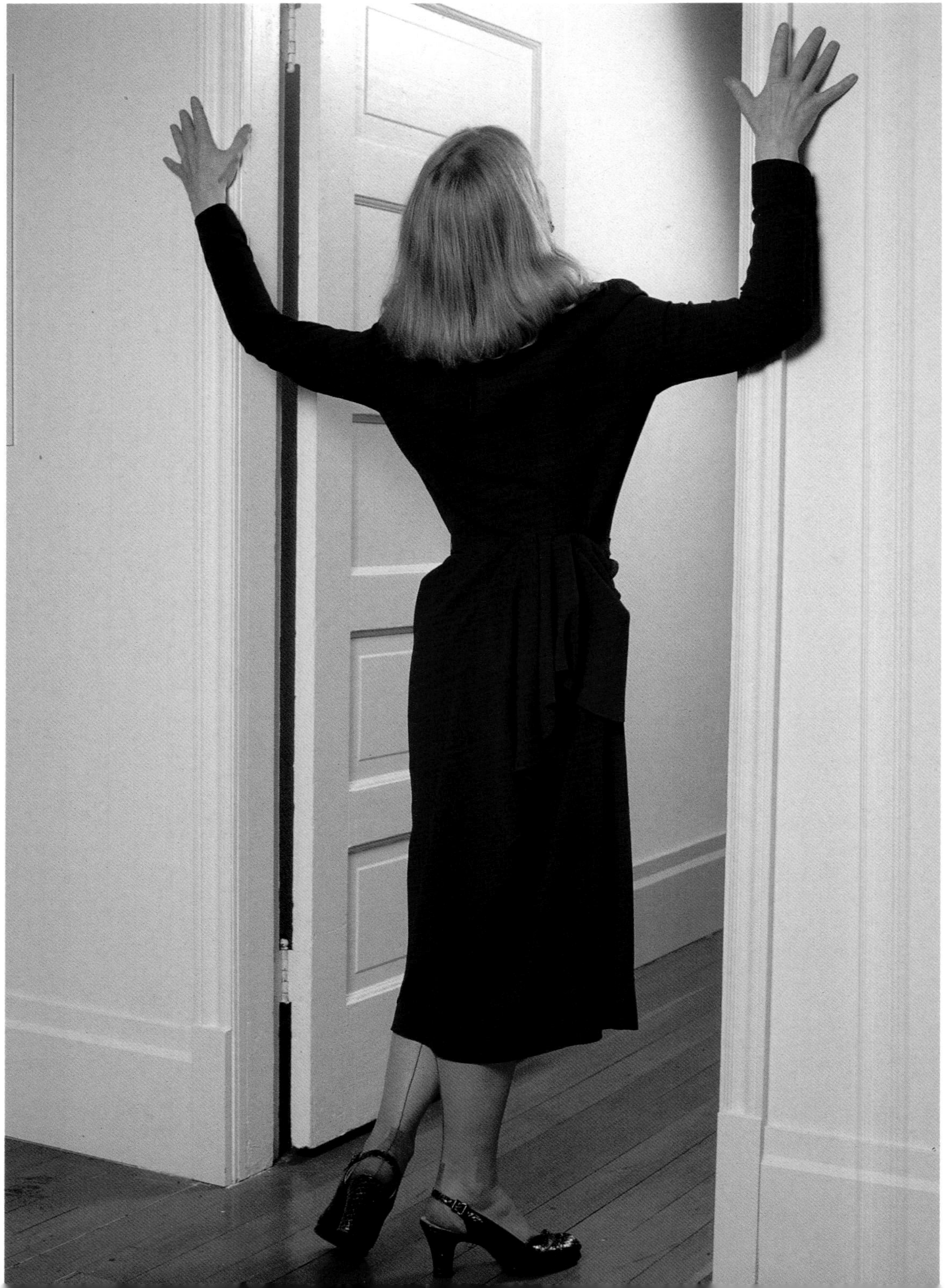

The War Years (1940-1946)

By 1940, it seemed inevitable that America would be drawn into the world fray. Just two years earlier, the war had erupted in Europe, where utility clothing was the fashion of necessity. This short, tailored look was often paired with sensible shoes like rocker clogs. Silk stockings were on the way out and ankle socks were on the way in!

Leather was scarce overseas, its use restricted to boots for soldiers. Old shoes were carefully polished and preserved under the Make Do and Mend campaign. This is also when fragile skins like crocodile and cobra were hauled out of storage by desperate shoe manufacturers and used for plain pumps and basic oxfords. It was a strange contrast of luxury and deprivation.

America did not enter the war until 1942 and then we were spared the ravages of bombing and battlefield. Even though Uncle Sam restricted the amount of fabric that could be used for clothing in Government Regulation L-38, our factories continued to produce leather shoes. Instead of silk, there were nylon stockings. But new shoes and sheer hose could not be obtained overseas, even with rationing coupons.

It was the blitzkrieg in Britain and the resistance in occupied France. The Brits kept a stiff upper lip and stomped about in brogues and clogs. For Parisians, gaiety of dress became a mark of pride, expressed with paper flowers and pipe-cleaner bows pinned to hat brims and shoe vamps.

The ubiquitous platform helped lift and lighten the look of utility clothing. Since wool was reserved for uniforms, women resorted to making over the civilian suits left behind by husbands and boyfriends. Hem lines went up, and shoulders went out. In jackets, peplums replaced draping. In skirts, gores and pleats were employed for ease of movement, rather than waste fabric by cutting on the bias. Altogether, it was a straight and boxy silhouette.

The wedgie is another 1940s classic. When the last stockpiles of leather were exhausted, European shoe designers were inspired to make cork-soled shoes. These were cut into a wedge shape for strength. The

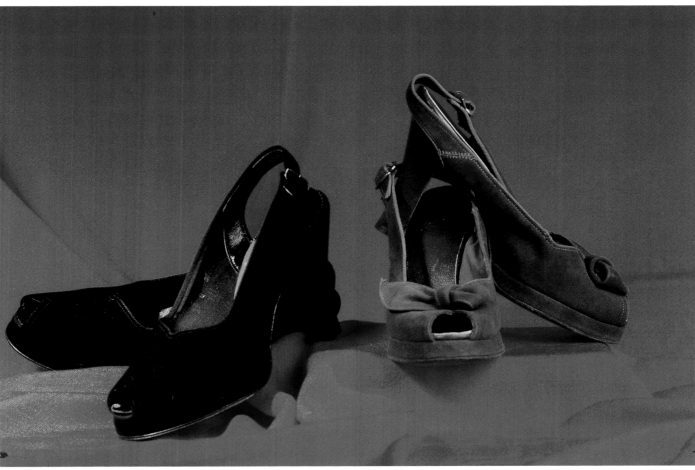

Like demitasse stirred with a silver spoon, these platforms from the mid-1940s are sophisticated, sweet, and strong. The pewter pair is by Marc Paul; the other designer is unknown. *Courtesy of Lottie Ballou.* Value: $45-65.

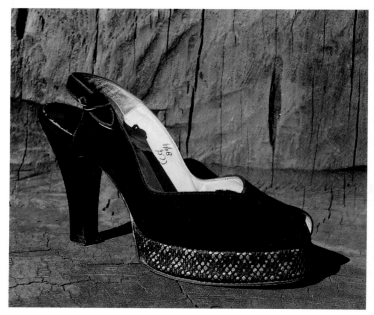

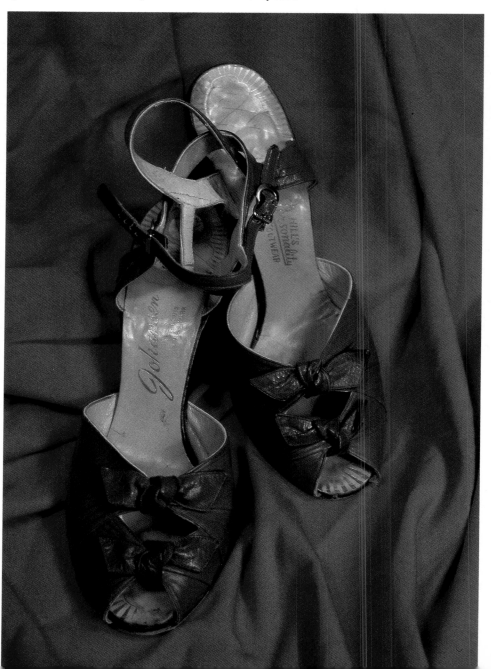

Below: A cluster of grape bows for a dance shoe, circa 1940–45, by Johansen. *Collection of Connie Beers.* Value: Special.

Above: Black lace in a stylized floral wraps the brilliant gold platform soles like a modish mantilla. Designed by Beleganti, circa 1949. *Courtesy of Deco Diva.* Value: $45-65.

Right: Cecil B. De Mille could not have done a better job casting these wedgies, in royal purple suede and queenly gold cobra. By Tweedies, for epic evenings in the mid-1940s. *Courtesy of Deco Diva.* Value: $75-95.

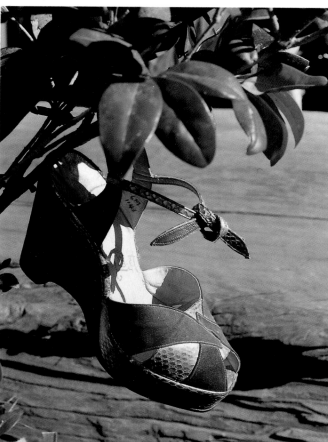

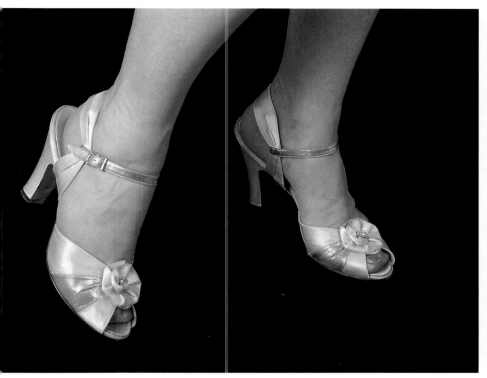

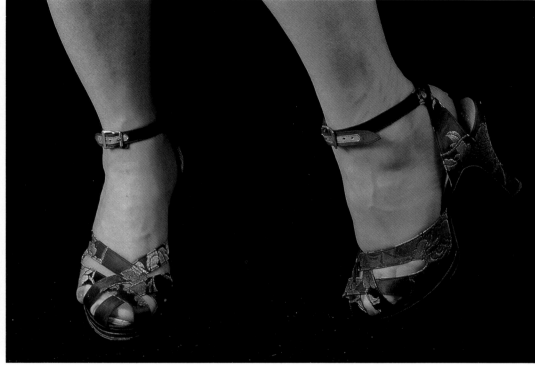

Creamy satin sandals with roses at the toes, for evening finery circa 1940. Courtesy of Barbara Grigg Vintage Fashion. Value: $55-75.

Silken strippy-strappy sandals in a regal brocade, circa 1945. *Courtesy of Barbara Grigg Vintage Fashions.* Value: $45-65.

uppers might be raffia, string, or braided scraps of fabric. The wedge itself might be covered to match or left bare. To relieve a slightly orthopedic look, wedgies were sometimes cut with a hole through the heel—nicknamed the loop, flying buttress, and doughnut.

When the soldiers were home on leave, women were glad to dress up. Silk might have been rationed and leather scarce, but festive shoes were still available in *faux* suede, rayon faille, and woven cellophane. Ankle-straps were popular, often combined with sling-back heels and platform soles. For trim, rhinestones or beads were prong-set into a platform sole and big bows were jauntily angled above a peep-toe.

For some collectors, there is no greater joy than finding mint-condition platforms, perhaps with Bakelite cherries clustered at the toe, or multi-colored rhinestones lighting up the ankle strap. Wedgies are another favorite and are relatively easy to find in casual straw and playful printed cottons.

The platform, wedge, and ankle-strap will forever be associated with this era. Bear in mind, however, that lissome shoes with slim heels were also widely available, and were especially stylish in the early '40s.

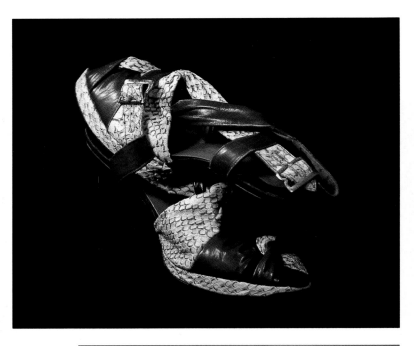

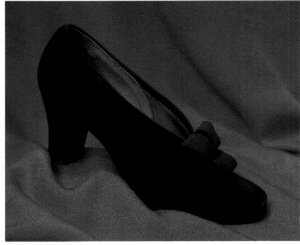

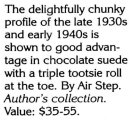

The delightfully chunky profile of the late 1930s and early 1940s is shown to good advantage in chocolate suede with a triple tootsie roll at the toe. By Air Step. *Author's collection.* Value: $35-55.

Above: Cocoa kid and cobra wrap around the foot and tie at the toe. These exotic platforms are by Peacock Shoes, circa 1945. Since reptile skin was unsuitable for combat boots, many shoes in the otherwise austere war years were fashioned from these luxury skins. *Courtesy of Luxe.* Value: $75-95.

Right: Two shades of suede leaves are illuminated in gold kid for a fancy pair of fall shoes from I. Miller, circa 1945. *Collection of Pamela Joyce.* Value: Special.

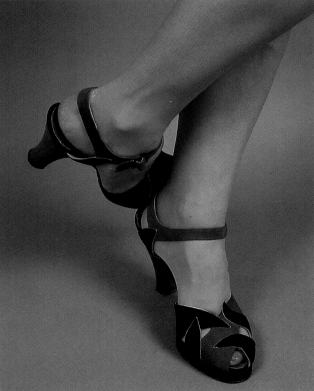

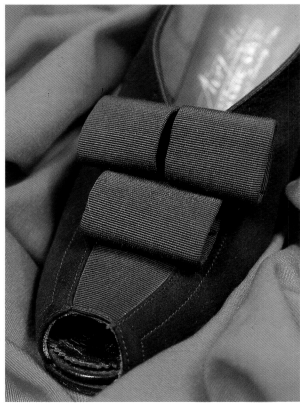

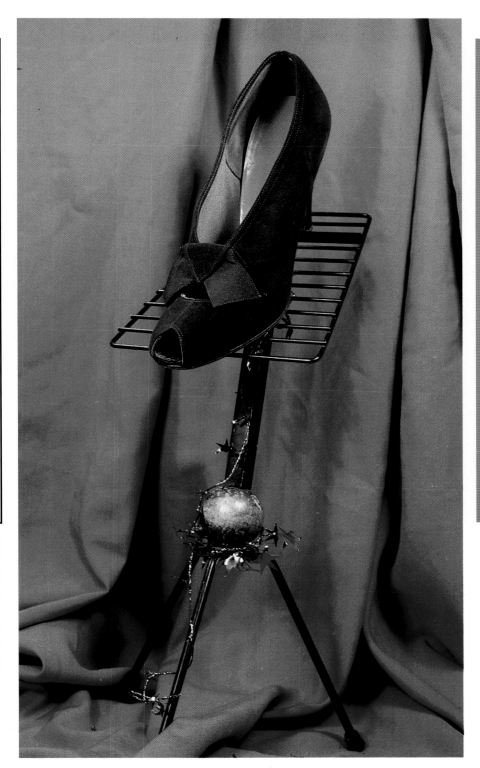

Above: It's September 1947, but the chubby 1930s profile is going strong, as seen in this advertisement for the label "twenty-ones" by the Barrett Shoe Co. The amusing green slingbacks are aptly named Jabot after a fluted double-ruff at the toe. These styles sold for $8.95 and $9.95.

Right: Another shoe in chocolate suede with a tailored grosgrain bow, from the late 1940s. Note the slimmer profile and higher heel, as compared to the tootsie roll pumps shown earlier on the previous page. *Author's collection.* Value: $25-35.

Within the advertisement:

To her new words are exciting... *Eleanor Kask*

young assistant to the president of Funk & Wagnalls, has the exciting job of promoting a brand new kind of dictionary—the New College Standard. Eleanor mirrors you, the fashion-wise young woman for whom we've created TWENTY-ONES.

JERRY

PERC

DRESS BY PEG NEWTON

you'll be exciting in

Twenty-ones

EXCITING FOOTWEAR

JABOT

"HALF-HIGHs"—the heel news of the year on TWENTY-ONES—the shoe news of the year. We have created glamorous pumps, sandals, dress shoes, and tailored shoes with this important new heel. Wear them— hear the raves! The name TWENTY-ONES is proudly stamped in gold in every pair. About $8.95, $9.95.

BARRETT SHOE CO., DIVISION OF GENERAL SHOE CORPORATION, NASHVILLE, TENN.

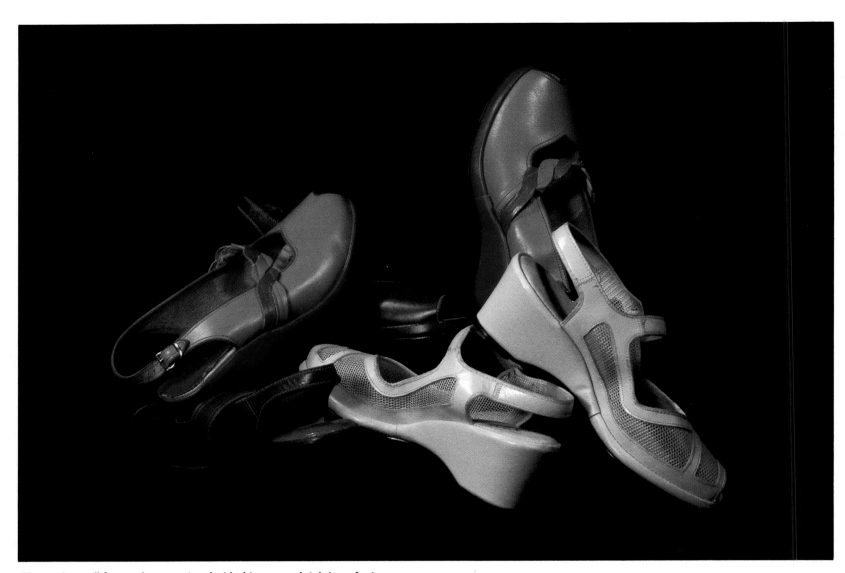

The wedgie will forever be associated with this era, and rightly so for it was a style spawned by the necessity of wartime. Faced with leather shortages, creative designers like Ferragamo and Perugia made soles from cork and balsa wood that were wedge-shaped for strength. The colorful trio shown here are all from the mid-1940s. *Courtesy of Lindy's Shoppe.* Value: $25-45 per pair.

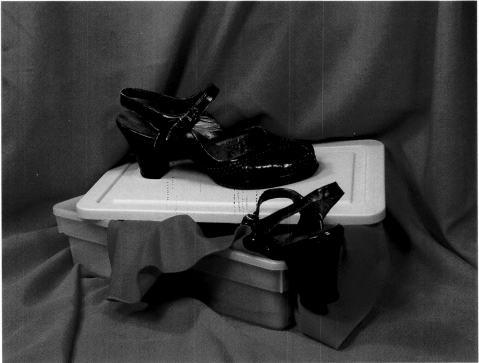

Left: Navy kid, so right for change-of-season dressing in the late 1940s. *Courtesy of Lottie Ballou.* Value: $35-55.

Below: Mesh inserts were a popular way to cool off tired feet, as seen in these two pair of navy shoes from the mid- to late-1940s. The city-wise pumps are by I. Miller, the countrified oxfords are by Hughes of New York. *Pumps from the Collection of Sheryl Birkner; oxfords courtesy of Luxe.* Value: $35-55.

High-steppers from the Naturalizer Fit Parade of 1947. The company motto was "the shoe with the beautiful fit." Each of these beauties sold for $6.95.

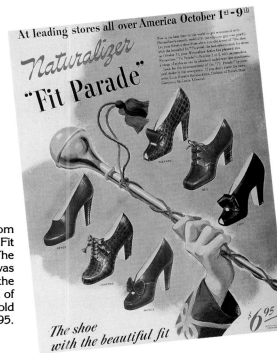

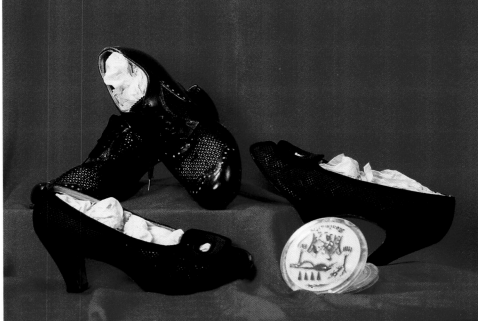

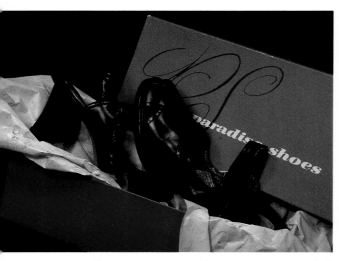

Above: Perky Paradise Shoes in shiny brown kid. These are new\old stock, shown in the original box, from the early 1940s. *Author's collection.* Value: $35-55.

Right: The post-war years were clearly a time of transition, in all walks of life, and that included shoe styles! Shown are brown suede dress pumps by Gayla, in a slimmer and simpler silhouette that would prevail after the New Look burst on the fashion scene in 1947. *Collection of Sheryl Birkner.* Value: $35-55.

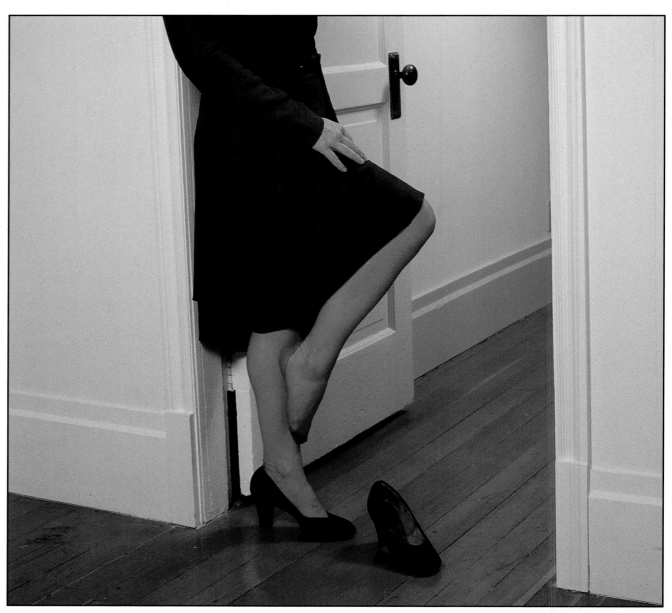

New and Newer Looks (1947–1956)

When Christian Dior launched his first collection in 1947, the chunky platforms and wedgies of the war years were swept away in a cloud of chiffon. For the next decade, the world followed every snip of Dior's scissors.

Skirts pouffed and belled, hem lines rose and fell, waistlines came and went, but the silhouette was always feminine. A new, simpler shoe was called for that would not distract from the "new look." Dior chose Roger Vivier, a fellow Parisian, to create an exclusive line of footwear to complement each collection.

It is almost impossible to overstate Dior's influence on clothing, and the same is true of Vivier's impact on shoe design. His basic *ouvre* was the pump, wherein he experimented with heel shapes like the *choc* and *comma*. For variety, Vivier mixed coarse linen or tweed, with smooth patent leather. For glamour, he used the finest brocade and silk jacquard, accented with a flawless jeweled button.

In the late 1940s and early '50s, the most elegant ensembles were accessorized with bold statement jewelry. On the head would be a hat that depended more on the line of its cut and the quality of its material than on trimming. On the feet were basic black suede pumps for day and strappy black silk sandals for night. The sides were cutaway, the toes were almond-shaped, and the vamps formed a gentle "V." This elegant silhouette rested on a delicate, gently curved, mid-height heel.

Above: Get ready for a garden party in the mid-1950s, in sprightly linen pumps with daffodil embroidery and spring-green spike heels. By Joseph Diamond. *Courtesy of Vintage Silhouettes.* Value: $25-35.

Right: Black and white tweed became trendy after Dior cut suits from his signature hound's-tooth check in the mid-1950s. *Courtesy of Barbara Grigg Vintage Fashion.* Value: $15-25.

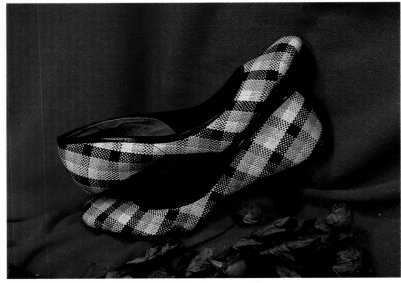

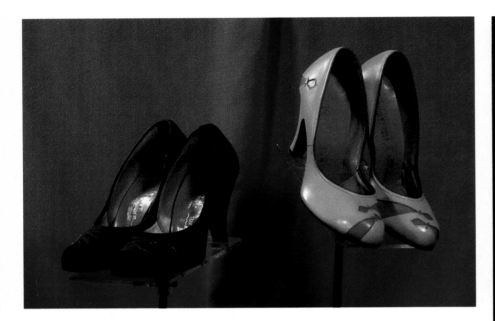

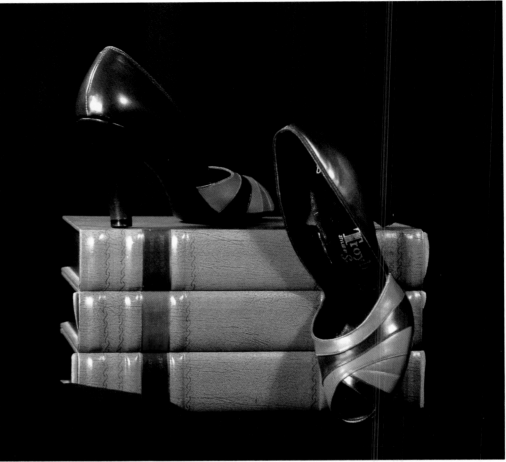

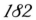

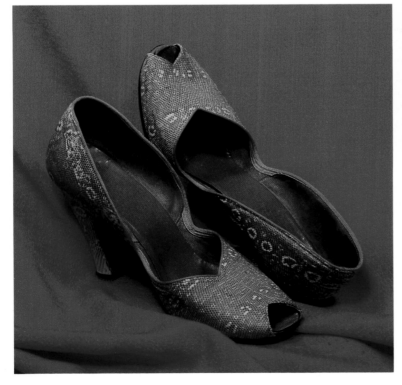

Above: The saffron and paprika binding on this stack of mock books is a perfect complement for the tri-color décolleté pumps. The shoes were designed by Seymour Troy for Troylings, circa 1955. *Courtesy of Luxe.* Value: $35-55.

Top left: These round-toed, high-heeled pumps are like reverse images in cream kid and caramel suede. From the mid-1950s by Parades (cream), and Pat Hagerty for Patricia Pat (caramel). *Courtesy of Lindy's Shoppe.* Value: $25-45.

Left: The décolleté instep, a vixenish look from the mid- to late 1950s, shown here in cobra. *Courtesy of Lottie Ballou.* Value: $35-55.

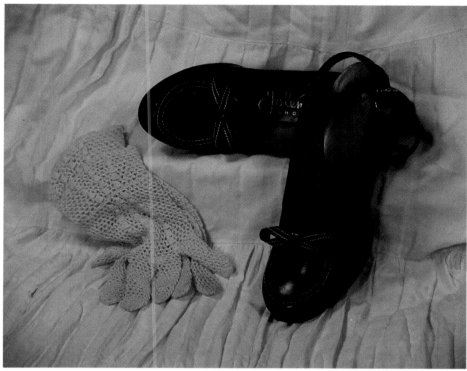

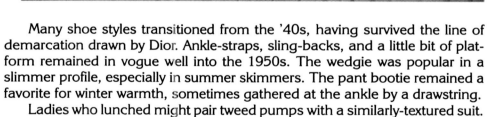

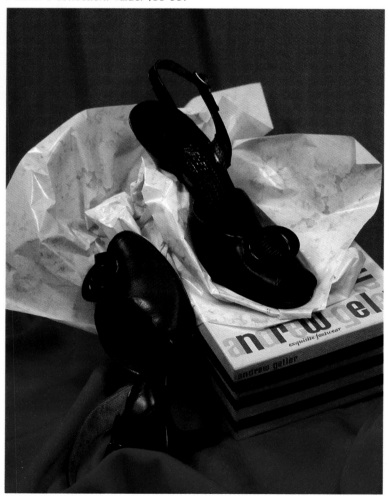

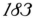

Left: A jaunty nut-brown leather slingback in new\old stock. This style, by Jolene, was perfect for a campus co-ed in the early 1950s. *Courtesy of Lindy's Shoppe.* Value: $25-45.

Below: Slingbacks with a groovy buckle. Crafted in fine fawn calfskin by Andrew Geller and shown in the original box, circa 1955. These late-day shoes were never worn, and were purchased from the extensive estate of a department store heiress in Sacramento. *Author's collection.* Value: $35-55.

Many shoe styles transitioned from the '40s, having survived the line of demarcation drawn by Dior. Ankle-straps, sling-backs, and a little bit of plat-form remained in vogue well into the 1950s. The wedgie was popular in a slimmer profile, especially in summer skimmers. The pant bootie remained a favorite for winter warmth, sometimes gathered at the ankle by a drawstring.

Ladies who lunched might pair tweed pumps with a similarly-textured suit. Working gals wore patent, suede, and kid pumps with shirtwaists and the new chemise. In the new suburbs, whether running errands in the station wagon or barbequeing in the backyard, the 1950s woman could be comfortable in Capri slacks and colorful canvas flats.

The pump still reigned in the mid-1950s, but it had grown slimmer, with an elongated toe and news-making stiletto heel. Platforms, wedgies, and ankle-straps were passé since they detracted from the desired "reed slim" look. The sides were no longer cut-away, but they might feature cut-outs. Sling-backs remained in style, especially for spring, and toes were "capped" after Coco Chanel made her couture comeback in the late '50s.

Within the discipline of a basic pump form, shoe designers relied on the color and quality of materials for a variety of looks and moods. For everyday there was patent leather, pleated suede, pearlized kid, exquisitely-wrapped raffia, and slubbed linen. For after-five it was silk-screened floral prints and radiant Thai silk. Gold kid was *soigné* for evening, often trimmed with glitter or rhinestones in the same gilded hue.

In color, shoes ran the rainbow, and were often perfectly matched to a dress or suit. Likewise, shoes were trimmed with dressmaker detailing like button-down tabs, fabric-covered buckles, and simple bows.

In 1954 the Oriental touch made a brief but vivid appearance in fashion and footwear. Look for harem-inspired mules with turned-up toes, evening pumps in silk the color and pattern of an obi sash, rattan-wrapped heels, and *faux* bamboo buckles.

The decade wound down with pumps and flats in neutral tones of leather, silk, and linen. Patrician shades of cream, oyster white, and beige were given some pizazz with an eggshell over glaze, and Easter-egg pastels were permanently shined with an overlay of vinyl. By 1957, the stiletto was cut-down for the low-slung look of a d'Orsay pump. At all times the bywords were elegance, sophistication, and suitability.

Seamless nylon stockings first appeared in the early '50s, but at first they were too baggy—much like tube stockings had been in the teens. For this reason, stylish women still wore seamed nylons until the late '50s when manufacturers finally learned how to fit nylon to the leg, with greater tensile strength. Then women fell in love with sheer hose in a range of light tints.

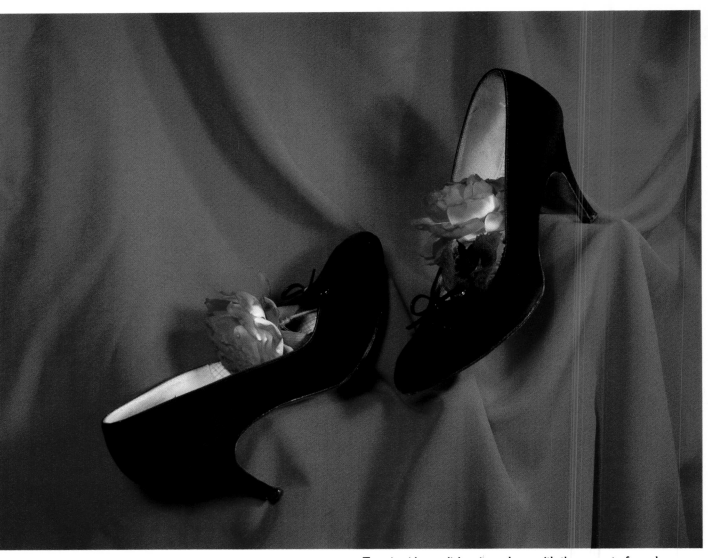

To pair with a stylish suit, perhaps with the accent of a red scarf at the throat. These brunette pumps in softest suede are tied at the leather-tip toe. By Fenton for Saks Fifth Avenue in the late 1950s. *Courtesy of It's About Time.* Value: $25-35.

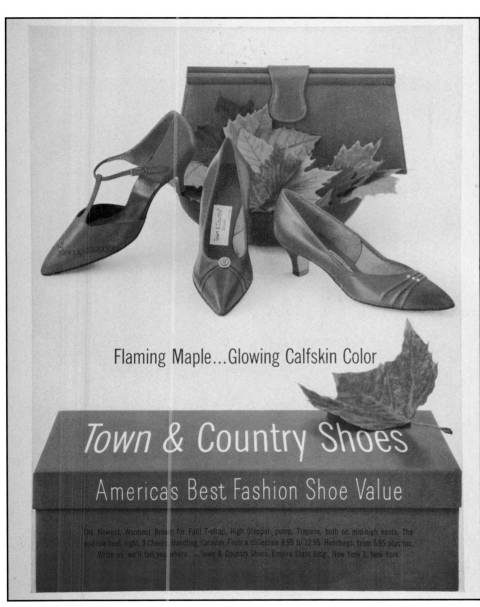

Flaming Maple...Glowing Calfskin Color

Town & Country Shoes

America's Best Fashion Shoe Value

The Newest, Warmest Brown for Fall! T-strap, High Stepper, pump, Trapeze, both on mid-high heels. The mid-low heel, right, 3 Cheers. Handbag, Caravan. From a collection 8.95 to 12.95. Handbags, from 5.95 plus tax. Write us, we'll tell you where... Town & Country Shoes, Empire State Bldg., New York 1, New York

Town & Country Shoes were geared to stylish young matrons in the suburban communities that sprouted up across America in the mid-1950s. Their gentrified look is exemplified in this trio of maple calfskin pumps, advertised in the September 1958 issue of *Vogue* magazine.

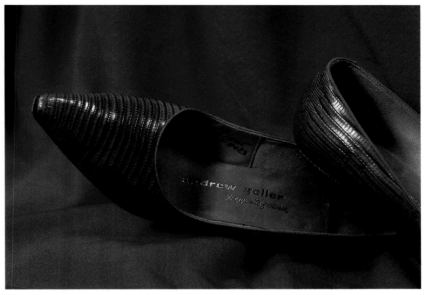

These fine-grained snakeskin pumps display a classic shape of the late 1950s. That debutante heel would soon skyrocket into a spike, then drop with a clunk. *Author's collection.* Value: $35-55.

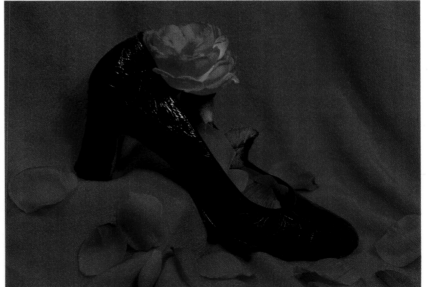
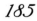

In the midst of changing hem lines and heel heights, many well-shod women opted for the conservative middle ground of basic pumps like these, in crocodile, for a note of luxury. *Author's collection.* Value: $34-65.

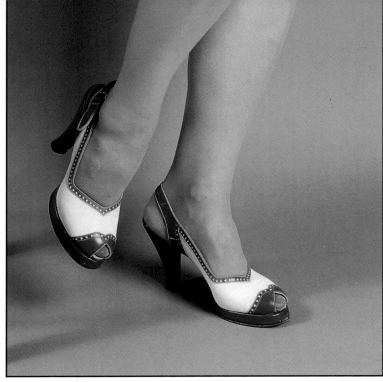

Slingback spectators with a peep-toe and perforated detailing, from the late 1940s or early 1950s. *Collection of Connie Beers.* Value: Special.

The casual chic of a spectator pump never had it so good as in the early 1950s. Jacqueline showed them in cream linen with burlap-brown kidskin, at the lower left of this advertisement from April 1950.

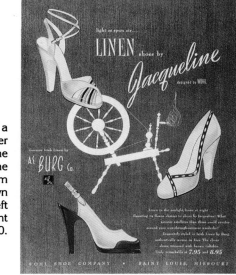

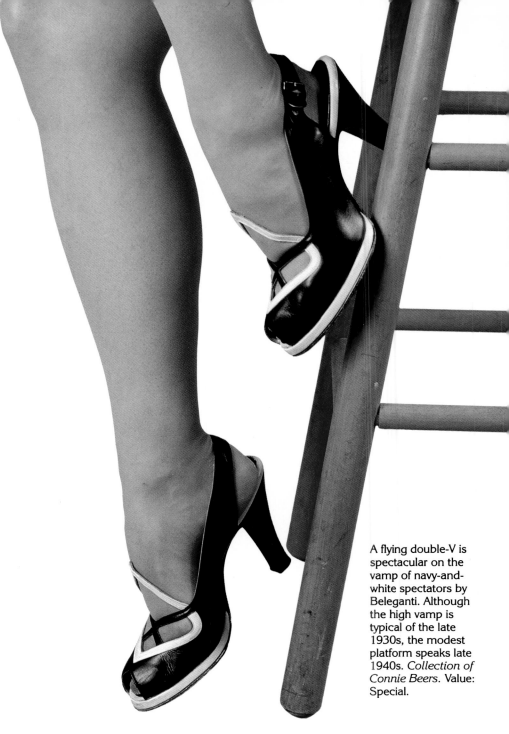

A flying double-V is spectacular on the vamp of navy-and-white spectators by Beleganti. Although the high vamp is typical of the late 1930s, the modest platform speaks late 1940s. *Collection of Connie Beers.* Value: Special.

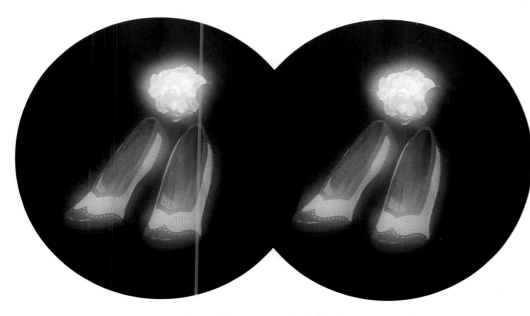

As seen through the spectator's field glasses, a pair of roan kid and cream net pumps circa 1955, by LifeStride. *Courtesy of It's About Time.* Value: $25-45.

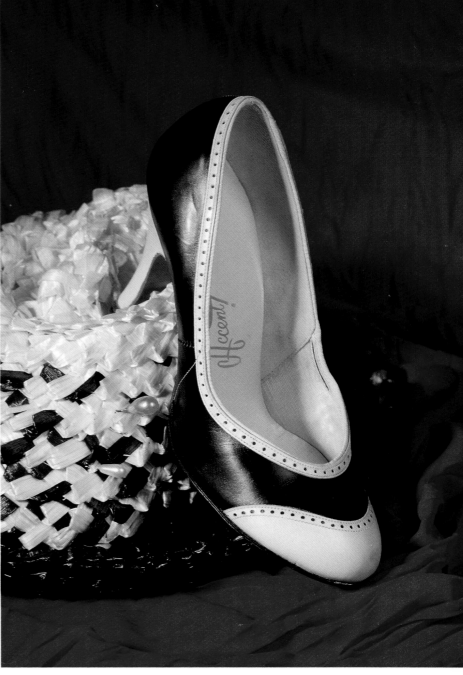

The traditional springtime spectator, a wardrobe staple circa 1959. By Accent, shown with a duotone straw toque by Mr. Arnold. *Collection of Connie Beers.* Value: Special.

Farewell to Elegance (1957–1962)

The lean and angular pump remained in style in these, the bridging years of two decades. It was the quintessential shoe for the shift in fashion that had been inspired by Dior and that would continue for many years after his death in 1957.

Dior's hand-picked successor was Yves St. Laurent, who had joined the couture house in 1955 at the incredibly young age of eighteen. In 1958, St. Laurent dazzled Paris with a brilliant first collection, including the radical "Trapeze Dress." It was a harbinger of breezy and youthful styles to come. That same year, Roger Vivier snipped off the tiptoe of his pumps for a new, if brief-lived, silhouette. This too was a forecast of the squared-toe shoes that would be paired with mini-dresses in the '60s.

These years saw a shift from the wasp-waist and padded hip of the New Look, to the hip-slung H-dress, the no-waist chemise, and the tent-shaped trapeze. The shoe silhouette relaxed in turn, moving from the steely stiletto to a low-slung d'Orsay. The form was still that of a pump and the emphasis was still on the quality of materials used in its construction. As before, there were gardens of silk-screened florals, sometimes sprinkled with rhinestones or glitter. Matched sets were the hallmark of a well-groomed woman, for day or evening.

For casual wear, there were sneakers and slip-in canvas flats. The ballerina flat was revived from the war years, as worn by Audrey Hepburn in the 1957 movie *Funny Face*. Flat leather sandals were cool for summer and were rendered chic in the gladiator motif from Bernardo of Italy. Wedgies returned for casual wear in raffia and colored straw for a "south of the border" fling and in brilliant jungle prints for a "south seas" theme.

Pool parties were a new and popular form of entertaining. Women wore hostess pajamas or caftans and gold kid sandals studded with *faux* stones. Soon rubber thongs would be worn pool side, embellished with plastic flowers to match a bathing cap.

This era is still wide-open for shoe collectors. Estate sales are just now coming on the market, opening the collections of women who purchased designer label shoes in the '50s. Stilettos, harem slippers, fiesta sandals, and patent leather prom heels would add zest to any collection.

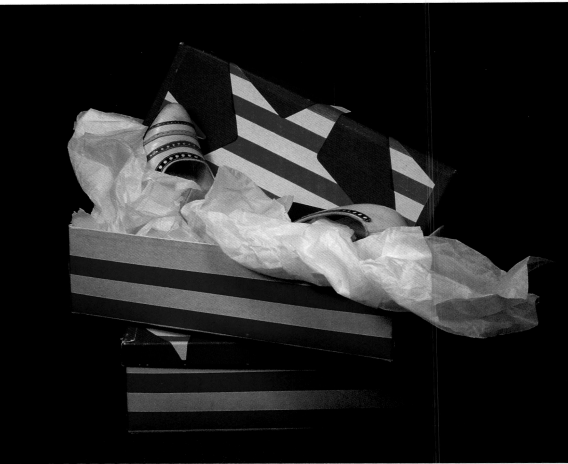

Miss America pumps in crayon colors banded on white, from the late 1950s. *Courtesy of It's About Time.* Value: $10-15.

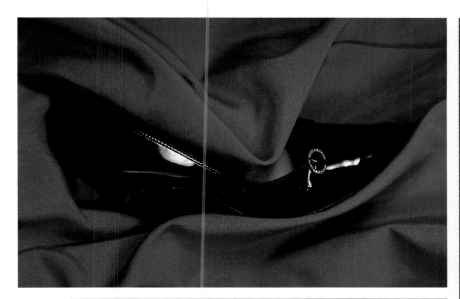

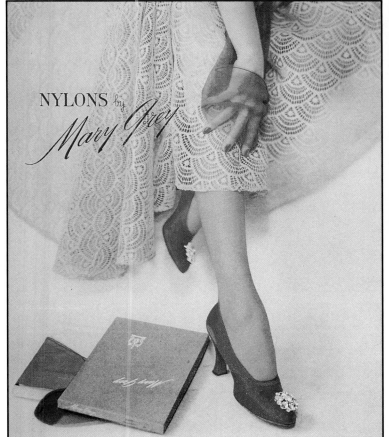

NYLONS *by Mary Grey*

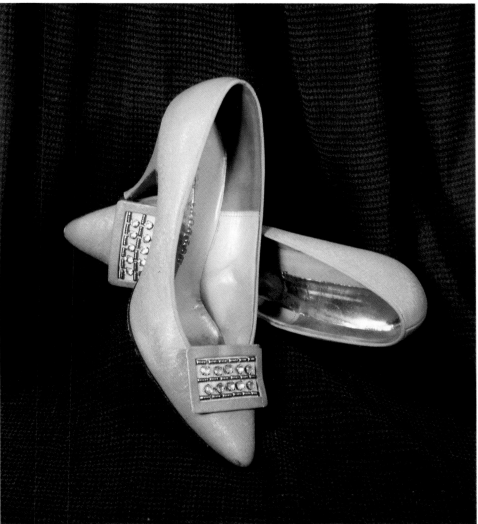

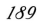

Above: Coquettish pumps whisper sweet nothings in baby blue, then flirt with bold buckles. All in a new-age rubberized fabric, from Herbert Levine circa 1959. *Collection of Gail Pocock.* Value: Special.

Above left: A low-slung black patent pump with princess heels and demure buckle trim. This style showed clothes to good advantage, with a touch of Audrey Hepburn's sprightly grace, circa 1957. *Courtesy of It's About Time.* Value: $10-15.

Left: Nylons were big business in the post-war years. The Mary Grey company emphasized the elegance of sheer hose, as seen in this ad from April 1950. The shoes are remarkable—baroque revival opera pumps with high, waisted heels, modernized by shocking pink satin and rhinestones twinkling from the toe, rather than the vamp.

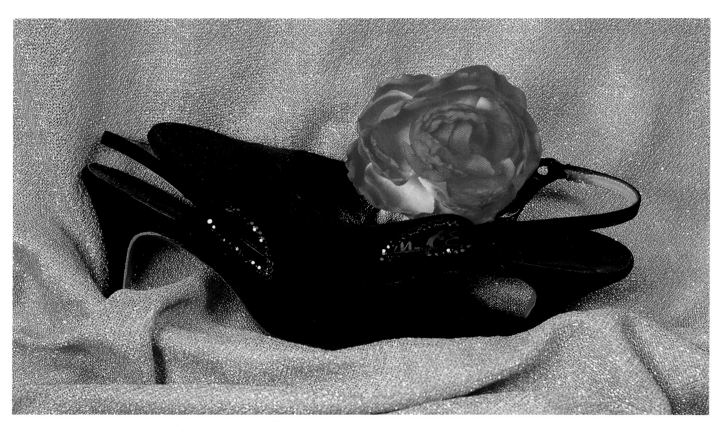

Mr. Easton styled these low-slung black silk evening shoes in the late 1950s. The teardrop cut-outs are outlined in faux marcasite. *Author's collection.* Value: $25-45.

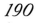

The harem heel, made famous by Taj Tajerie in the late 1950s, here interpreted in wood. Gold kid trim and a see-through vinyl vamp add more glamour. From Island Slippers, Made in Hawaii. *Courtesy of It's About Time.* Value: $25-35.

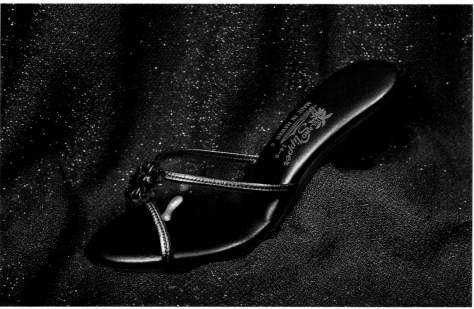

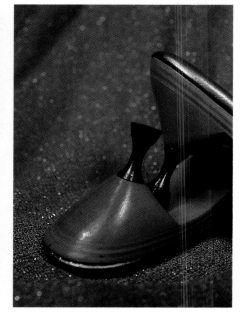

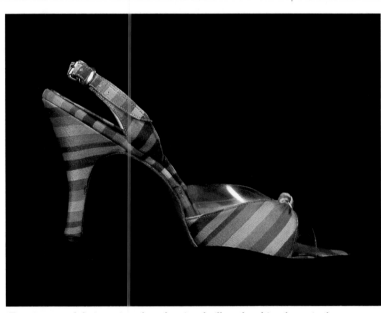

Evening sandals in striated and striped silk, edged in clear vinyl, from the mid-1950s. *Courtesy of It's About Time.* Value: $10-15.

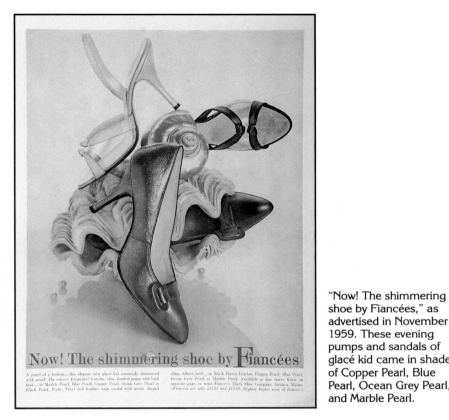

Now! The shimmering shoe by Fiancées

A jewel of a fashion...this elegant, new glacé kid seemingly shimmered with pearl! The colors? Exquisite! *Concha*: slim, banded pump with high heel...in Marble Pearl, Blue Pearl, Copper Pearl, Ocean Grey Pearl or Black Pearl. *Perla*: Vinyl and leather strip sandal with newly-shaped sling, stiletto heel...in Black Patent Leather, Copper Pearl, Blue Pearl, Ocean Grey Pearl or Marble Pearl. Available at fine stores listed on opposite page, or write Fiancées, Clark Shoe Company, Auburn, Maine. *(Fiancées are only $12.95 and $13.95. Slightly higher west of Denver.)*

"Now! The shimmering shoe by Fiancées," as advertised in November 1959. These evening pumps and sandals of glacé kid came in shades of Copper Pearl, Blue Pearl, Ocean Grey Pearl, and Marble Pearl.

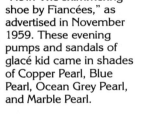

Pearlized plum pumps from De Liso Debs, circa 1955. *Courtesy of Lindy's Shoppe.* Value: $35-55.

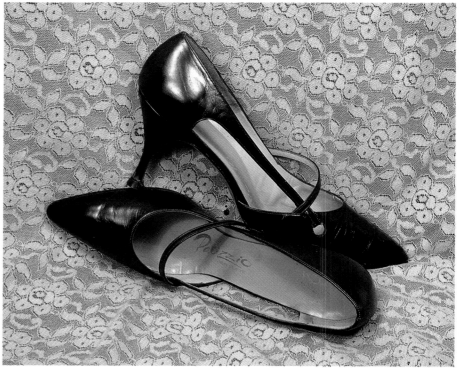

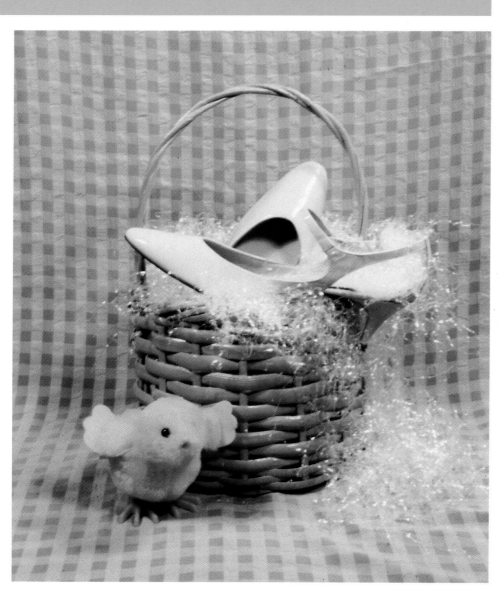

Above: More pearlized pumps, the color of folding money, by Palizzio. The cut-out insteps were a fad in the late 1950s and early 1960s. *Author's collection.* Value: $15-25.

Left: Perfect first heels for a young miss, circa 1959. In Easter-egg-pink patent, by Foot Flairs. *Courtesy of It's About Time.* Value: $15-25.

Age of Aquarius (1963–1975)

And the beat goes on! By the mid-1960s it was a mod, mod world as designers scrambled to gain back the market share that had steadily eroded after the overnight sensation of street-wise British designers like Mary Quant, Ossie Clark, Marion Foale, and Sally Tuffin. The in-look was all about linear lines, bold colors, and graphic patterns.

By now the so-called fine arts had permanently crossed the fashion barrier. Think Emilio Pucci, Andy Warhol, Zandra Rhodes, and Sonia Rykiel. Clothing designers were inspired by American op art, and its French cousin *trompe l'oiel*. Indeed, it seemed as if life imitated art in the inspired team of Rudy Gernreich and his model *cum* muse, Peggy Moffit. He contributed to the patterned stocking look with tights that matched the fabric of a mini-dress and body dress neck-to-toe stretch jersey. Moffit chose simple flats or demi-heel pumps to set off his "total look." (She went barefoot, of course, to model the notorious topless bathing suit that earned Gernreich the cover of *Time* magazine in 1964.)

Fashion was also influenced by visions of the space age, given that Sputnik had launched in 1957 and Neil Armstrong walked on the moon in 1969. White vinyl and clear plastic were a calling card for André Courreges, who showed his first collection in 1964. When he designed flashy go-go boots in these materials, they became a fashion icon for emancipated womanhood.

Large metallic sequins and disks were strung together by Paco Rabanne, a bright new star in the fashion firmament of 1966. He forged shifts and skirts that looked like suits of armor for new age Martians, shown with silver-kid flats and clear vinyl pumps. In keeping with this hard-edged look, Vivier designed thigh-high boots in silver vinyl and black knit with silver appliqué.

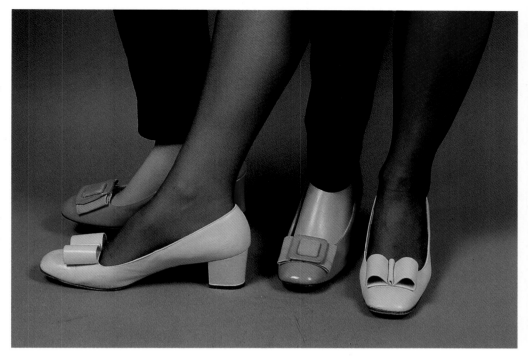

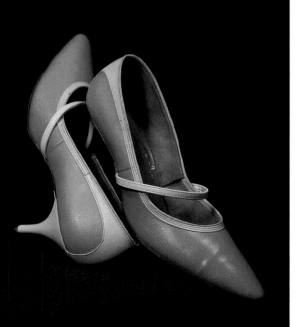

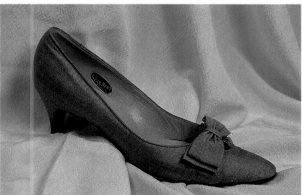

A low-slung debutante silhouette in lime green silk by WearBest. Imported from Hong Kong, circa 1967. *Author's collection.* Value: $15-25.

Above: Citrus colors were cool, and the glow of patent was hot. Seen here in low pumps, perfect with bold tights and mini-skirts. *Courtesy of It's About Time.* Value: $15-25.

Left: Sunshine colors cut a girlish figure on pumps styled for a youthful market. By Qualicraft, circa 1960. *Courtesy of It's About Time.* Value: $15-25.

193

Barbara Hulanecki designed exclusively for her innovative Biba boutique. She showed romantic styles in lace and velvet with a variety of historical references, from Renaissance to Victorian. Her clothing paired well with velvet ballet slippers, ribbon-tied ghillies, and embroidered suede boots. Betsey Johnson styled baby dolls and prairie dresses in smocked and ruffled cotton, anchored by Mary Janes and granny boots. Mary Quant launched a line of A-line shifts and tunics in oversized graphic prints and crayon colors, shown with patent leather T-straps.

The mods of London overlapped the hippies of San Francisco for further variety in style. Flower power might mean a stylized Quant daisy or a tie-dye skirt and macramé vest, worn with buffalo-hide, toe-ring sandals. The fashion byword of the 1960s was nothing if not eclectic .

It was a confluence of futuristic vision, historical drama, patty-cake and dress-up, and period revivals from Gibson Girl to the Andrews Sisters. These were boutique clothes, but they inspired instant knock-offs that were mass merchandised through department stores and catalogs. Even Barbie®, the beloved teenage fashion model, got a new wardrobe complete with vinyl mini-skirts and flowered bell-bottoms.

Eventually, the *haute couture* responded to the same design influences that had launched the boutiques. Emilio Pucci patterned silk pajamas and caftans were paired with jeweled toe-ring sandals, in the late '50s. Pierre Cardin cut angular clothes from bonded synthetics and his models glided down the runway in glacé silk ankle-boots, in the early '60s. St. Laurent created a new shoe classic in 1962 with his silver-buckled pilgrim. Some ten years later, he showed a Russian collection with fabulous fur-cuffed boots.

Hemlines had been steadily rising until the mini-skirt was launched in 1968. The emphasis was on leg, and lots of it. Whether from modesty or wind-chill, shorter skirts spawned a craze for richly patterned and thickly textured hosiery. It was white lace hose or glittery fishnet tights for evening, depending on whether a costume referenced "inner child" or outer space. Creamy crochet hose and black fishnet were worn during the day, contrasted with pastel kid heels or bright patent leather flats.

Pantyhose became an overnight sensation when launched in the early '70s. Until then, even trim young girls wore panty girdles under A-line skirts and shift dresses. They were necessary for one purpose only, which was holding hose to garter!

194

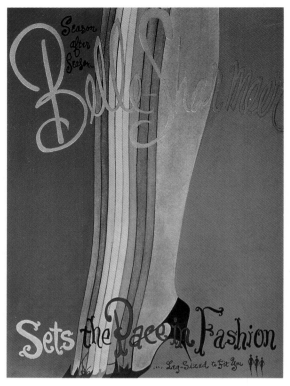

Left: As the decade of the 1950s drew to a close, designers began experimenting with the unexpected use of bold color in all manner of products, from bed linens to hosiery. As shown in this charming ad from 1960, Belle Sharmeer kicked off a rainbow chorus line for the long-of-limb and young-at-heart.

Below: Black patent pants boots, with *trompe l'oiel* spats in white kid. A playful fashion statement from the mid-1960s. *Courtesy of The Blue Parrot.* Value: $15-25.

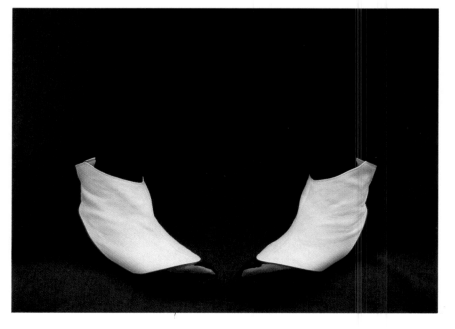

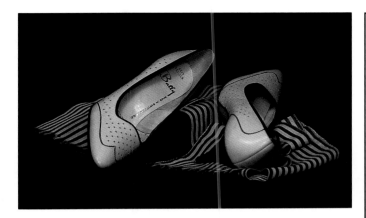

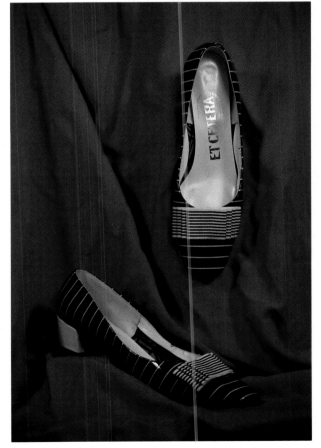

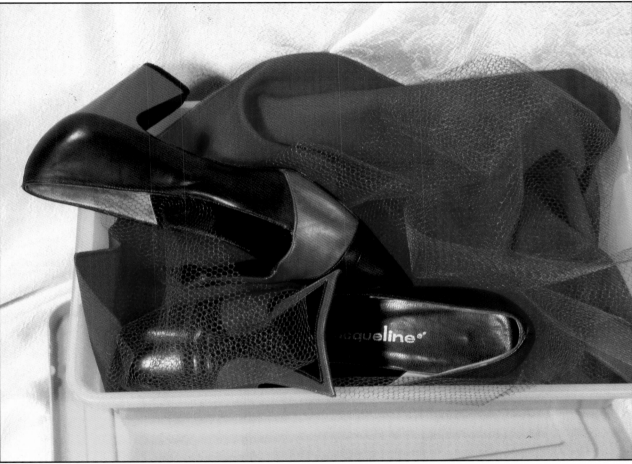

Above: Even everyday clothes had an element of costume drama in the 1960s, like these variations on the high-tongued courtier shoes of the Baroque period. In navy and red kid, by Jacqueline. *Courtesy of It's About Time.* Value: $15-25.

Above left: High-button shoes are revived, in a pancake-heel ankle-boot, the profile that was made popular by Courreges. Tucked inside is a bow-tied slingback by Marquise. *Boots courtesy of Luxe; slings courtesy of Lindy's Shoppe.* Value: boots, $35-45; slings, $15-25.

Left: Spectator pumps are classy in white kid and black patent, styled by Bally in the early 1960s. *Courtesy of Lindy's Shoppe.* Value: $25-35.

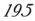

Boots were worn everywhere and in all seasons. They created a kicky, leggy, and adventurous look for the "sexy sixties." Platforms and rounded toes were popular for boots, an expansive volume that balanced the mid-calf midi-skirt of 1969. The midi was slit in front or back for ease of movement and a flash of outrageous boots in dyed cobra, patchwork leather, and embroidered suede. By the mid-1970s, the classic profile of the pump reappeared on a demi-platform sole with blocky high heels and squared-off toes.

Throughout this youth-quake era, there were still women *d'une certain age* who would not abandon the couture. These ladies turned to Givenchy, Halston, Norell, Blass, and Beene for styles that were youthful but not girlish. Their look was exemplified by Jackie Kennedy

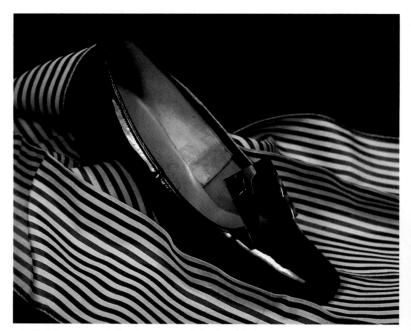

A slightly more subdued version of the buckled courtier pump, in black patent. From the late 1960s, by Risqué. Value: $15-25. *Courtesy of It's About Time.*

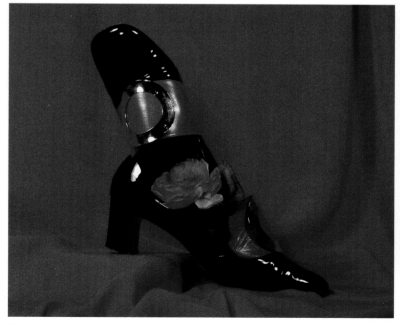

Another high-tongued shoe, this time in black and red patent, by Risqué. *Courtesy of It's About Time.* Value: $15-25.

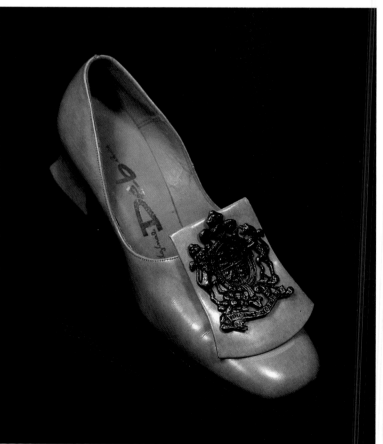

The courtier shoe, with a nod to the Brits. The heraldic buckle shouts Buckingham Palace and whispers Carnaby Street. *Courtesy of It's About Time.* Value: $15-25.

196

during her years in the White House, so aptly captured by Oleg Cassini in his autobiographical *100 Days of Magic*. She wore simply-cut clothes in luxury fabrics with her ubiquitous pillbox hat and classic mid-heel pumps.

Part of the fun in collecting shoes of the 1960s and 1970s is in discovering the range of styles and the mix of materials. Rubber, plastic, paper, cellophane, wood, and metal were combined in fantastic new forms, from one playful extreme to another. Also, there's always the possibility of finding bargains in a designer shoe since many women toss these shoes aside during periodic closet cleanings. You won't find Courrege boots or Vivier pumps this way, but you should be on the lookout for Delman, De Liso, and David Evins.

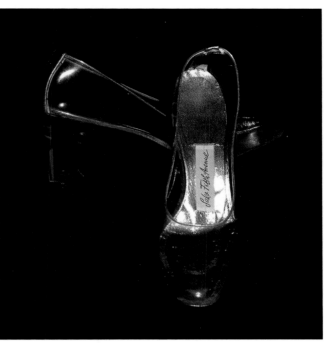

Left: These clearly cool Lucite pumps sold at Saks Fifth Avenue under the boutique label Beth's Bootery. They are attributed to Beth Levine, whose husband Herbert Levine designed a strikingly similar pair of low-heeled Lucite pumps with open-toe and slingback, also in the mid-1960s. *Courtesy of Luxe.* Value: $35-55.

Below: The illusion of a hologram in shimmering, iridescent vinyl. This is a good example of the way designers were experimenting with new materials during the 1960s and 1970s. Imported from London by Thos. Cort, Ltd. *Collection of Pamela Joyce.* Value: Special.

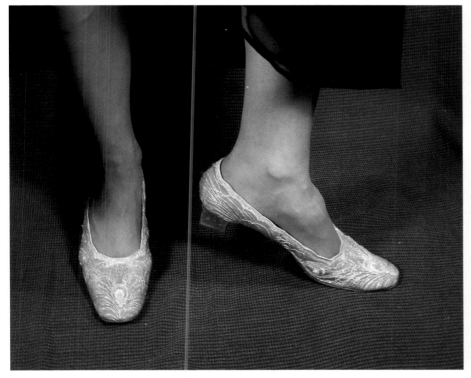

Arts and crafts made fashion headlines in the mid-1960s. Shoe designer Frank More echoed that trend in pumps that have the look of handmade lace. *Courtesy of Lottie Ballou.* Value: $25-35.

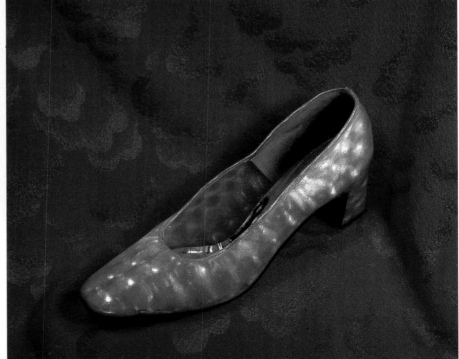

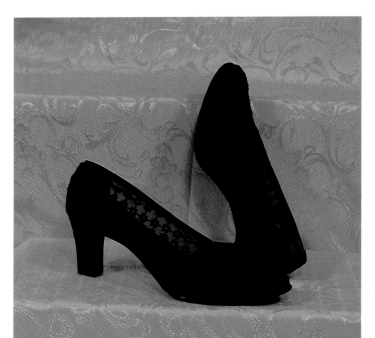

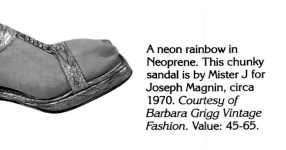

A neon rainbow in Neoprene. This chunky sandal is by Mister J for Joseph Magnin, circa 1970. *Courtesy of Barbara Grigg Vintage Fashion.* Value: 45-65.

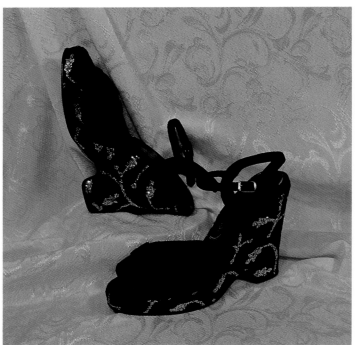

Above: Sedate black *poie de soie* and net pumps. For the mature woman, with a hint of "flower child" peeping out, in the stylized daisy motif used for the netting. By Fenton for Saks Fifth Avenue, circa 1965. *Courtesy of It's About Time.* Value: $25-35.

Right: Glittery fireworks spray across the wedge heels of dazzling black velvet sandals by Lady Carrie, circa 1969. This is, of course, a revival from the 1940s. Value: $35-55. *Courtesy of It's About Time.*

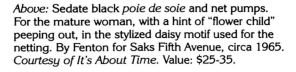

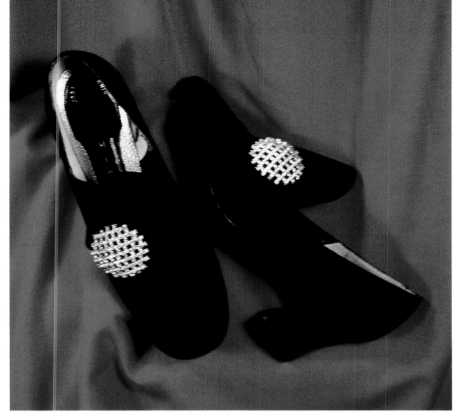

Left: A rhinestone latticework button is oversized for emphasis. It twinkles against striated black silk on a pair of high-tongued dress pumps, from the early 1970s. The label is Mister J for Joseph Magnin. *Courtesy of Cheap Thrills.* Value: $25-45.

Below left: One cabochon makes a gutsy fashion statement, on black satin pumps by Young Elite for Saks Fifth Avenue. The "crystal ball" look was also big in rings and earrings in the early 1970s. *Courtesy of It's About Time.* Value: $25-35.

Below: Faux topaz rings around a bold buckle that complements the color and texture of rich brown court shoes. By David Evins for I. Magnin. *Author's collection.* Value: $45-65.

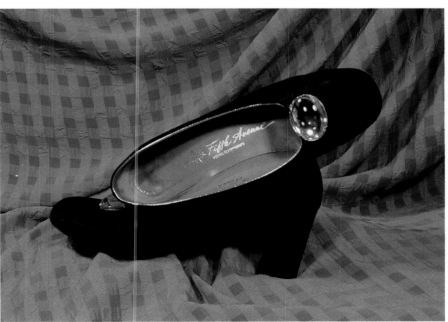

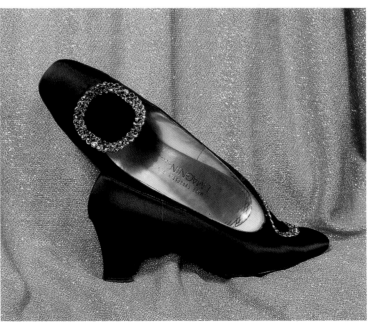

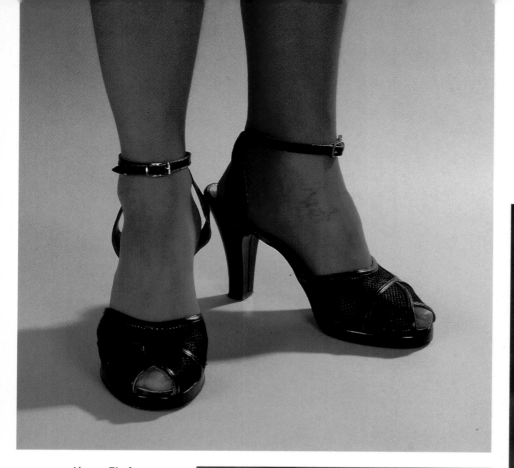

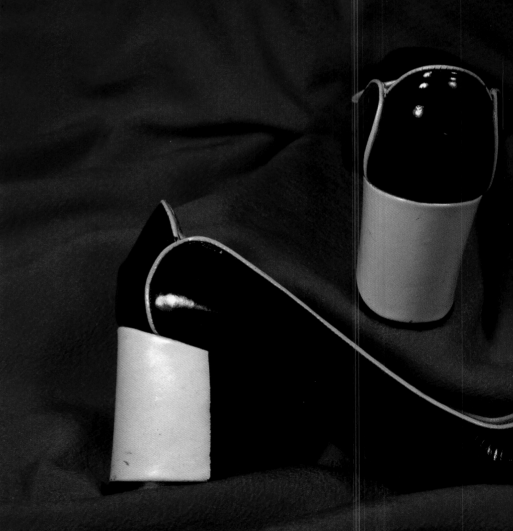

Above: Platforms were a major revival in the late 1960s, shown here in navy kid. Likewise, the mesh inserts and ankle straps are a revival of mid-1940s style, by QualiCraft. *Courtesy of It's About Time.* Value: $25-45.

Right: Black suede for a black-tie event, with not much left to the imagination. From the mid-1960s, by Sommer & Kaufman. *Courtesy of Barbara Grigg Vintage Fashion.* Value: $45-65.

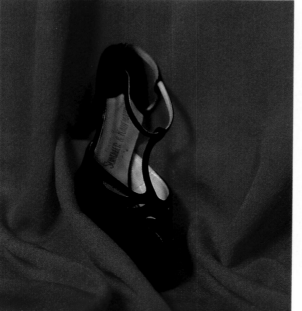

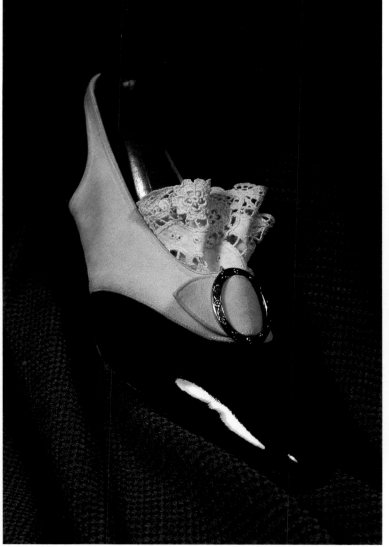

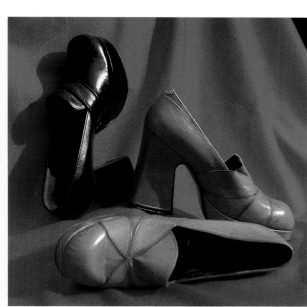

Chunky toes and clunky platform soles—two pair of pumps with all the awkward charm of puppy paws. These are new/old stock, in navy and luggage leather. They were styled for the adolescent set, circa 1975. *Courtesy of The Blue Parrot.* Value: $35-55.

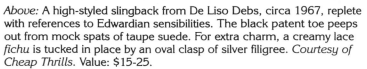

Above: A high-styled slingback from De Liso Debs, circa 1967, replete with references to Edwardian sensibilities. The black patent toe peeps out from mock spats of taupe suede. For extra charm, a creamy lace *fichu* is tucked in place by an oval clasp of silver filigree. *Courtesy of Cheap Thrills.* Value: $15-25.

Left: These pumps delight with the style contrast of curves and squares and the color fun of licorice and nougat. In patent leather by the *D'amica* label, an Italian import from the mid-1970s. *Courtesy of Cheap Thrills.* Value: $25-45.

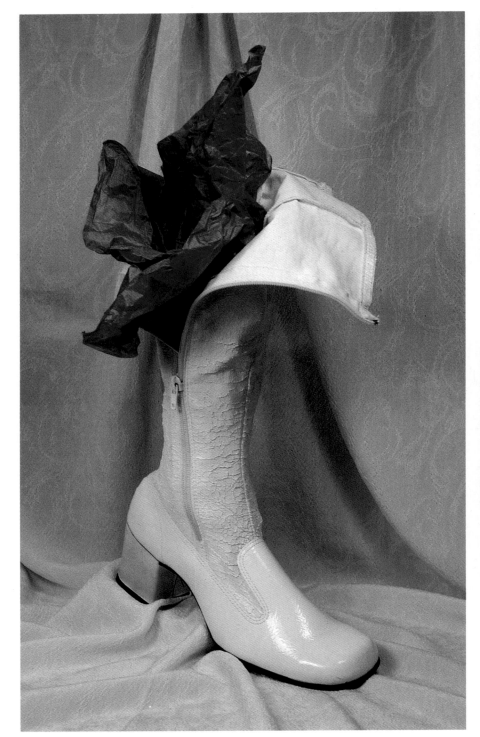

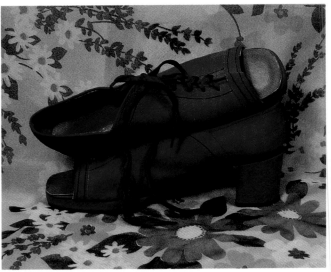

Hot pink suede sandals, laced up the instep like a *bustier*. They are so tacky, they bypass poor taste and emerge as an art form. *Courtesy of Lottie Ballou.* Value: $25-35.

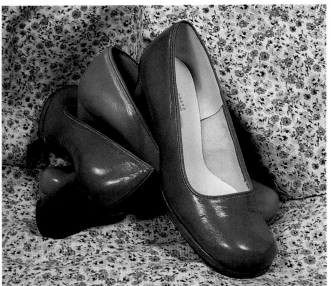

Above: Snub-toed platform pumps in lime green and turquoise leather. Both pair are new\old stock by Miss America, from the mid-1970s. *Courtesy of It's About Time.* Value: $25-45.

Left: These go-go boots feature elasticized vinyl uppers to hug the calf like a second skin. They're the worse for wear—with hot pants, during the summer of 1969. *Author's collection.* Value: Special.

Chapter IX

CARE AND STORAGE

Given the frantic pace at which many of us live today, it may seem fussy or even archaic to be concerned about the gloss of a patent toe or the nicety of a heel lift. Paradoxically, the attention to detail and devotion to ritual, that is required for proper shoe care, can bring a soothing sense of contentment to an otherwise harried day. It may be that the busy process of polishing and mending so engages the hands that it frees the mind to sort out the tangles and tensions of modern life.

The crackle of new tissue paper and the sweet scent of sachet turn the simple act of storing vintage shoes into an experience at once innocent and sensual, and ultimately satisfying.

From sad experience, the author cautions that alligator, crocodile, cobra, and similar reptile skins become especially brittle with age. They split along the same lines that formed their beautiful patterning. Be sure your vintage shoes are supple before you wear them, since once the skin splits there is no means of repair. A good shoe shop can glue the skin in place for display or storage, but they can't be worn again.

Spit 'n' Polish

The sheen of highly-polished leather was long a hallmark of the gentleman, and the professional pride of his valet. In England, there developed the rather esoteric practice of "boning" shoes. The bone was usually the shank of an elk or deer, which have the proper osseous texture and natural oil deposits to create a lustrous finish on leather. Several times a year, the valet would apply a base wax and then gloss it to a fine, subdued patina by rubbing with the shoe bone. The process could take half an hour, yet it was considered time well spent in the pursuit of sartorial excellence.

Diana Vreeland, the wealthy socialite who later became an arbiter of fashion through her editing roles at *Harper's Bazaar* and *Vogue*, recalled that her father's valet would bone his shoes for six months before they were deemed fit to wear, using, no less, an exotic rhinoceros horn. She followed in his footsteps, insisting that her lady's maid use the same type of horn, not only on the uppers but on the soles as well. "Why, I wouldn't *dream* of wearing shoes with unpolished soles. I mean, you go out to dinner and suddenly you lift your foot and the soles aren't impeccable ... what could be more ordinary?" Words to live by!

During the Directoire period in the late 1700s, and again during the mid-1800s, women wore extremely thin-soled shoes. This was also when a waltz craze swept Europe, and it was commonplace for popular girls to bring an extra pair—they could wear through the soles of new slippers, in the course of a ball! This bit of fashion trivia certainly gives new meaning to the *Twelve Dancing Princesses* fairytale.

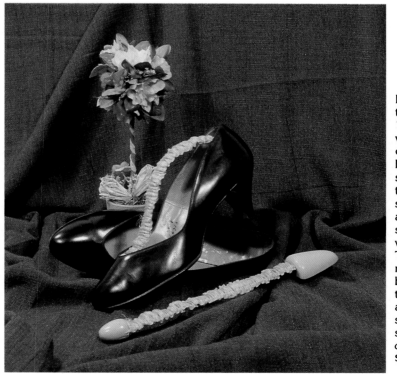

In the 1920s through the 1960s, fashionable women took good care of their leather pumps with shoetrees like these. A similar, sturdier variety was available for shaping boots and walking shoes. These flexible metal trees are still being made, but the vintage variety are nicer with their shirred ribbon sleeves. *Author's collection.* Value: $10-15.

We can take a tip from the boys, who received meticulous advice about the proper care of leather shoes in *Esquire*. The following article "Footnotes to a Summer Shoe Wardrobe" ran in 1934:

"The picture tells the story of the various shoes but the matter of their care is a story in itself. First, it is almost as important to tree your shoes, upon retiring, as it is to remove them. Next (unless you have a valet—and aren't we all?) you must clean them. To take the new look off brown calf shoes, vary the shade of polish—a dark brown one day and a deep red, like the famous Royal Navy Dressing, the next. After applying polish, brush, then rub in Meltonian Cream, then polish the shoes briskly. White and white trimmed shoes require a liquid paste that won't rub off. To get a high shine on white buckskin, use Coates Polish on Turkish toweling, let dry, then rub with soft cloth. Contrary to what you hear, don't use a wire brush on brown buckskin, use an old hairbrush. Coat the edges of soles and heels with black waterproof enamel. Clean the leather trimming on white shoes with a neutral Meltonian Cream."

On a more practical note, here are some basic tips gleaned from housewives, personal maids, and valets. They are reliable receipts from a well-run home in days gone by:

• Sprinkle a hefty tablespoon of bicarbonate of soda into each shoe and leave overnight, to eliminate odor.

• For stiff leather, stuff each shoe with a peeled, raw potato cut into chunks. Left overnight, the leather will again be pliable.

• Rejuvenate grubby suede with a light sanding. Take care to use the finest grade of sandpaper (00). Then, rub the shoes all over with a cloth lightly wet with vinegar.

• For a mirror finish on patent leather, try rubbing the shoes with raw onion then buffing with an absorbent dry cloth.

• Fine leather responds to a mask of raw egg white. Leave it on until dry, then wipe it off and buff it up with a soft cotton cloth.

• For bald spots on suede shoes, gently rub with the finest grade of sandpaper (00) to raise the nap. Or steam the bald spot by holding it over a boiling teakettle, then gently brush up the nap with a soft toothbrush.

204

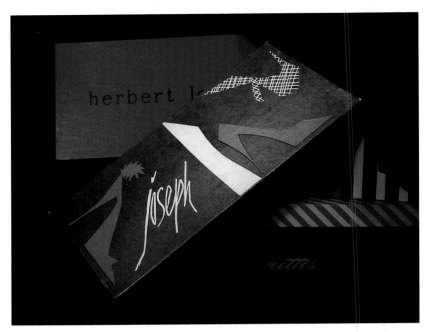

Shoeboxes stack readily for storage. These are by well-known designers of the 1960s. The value of boxes from the mid-century is negligible. With a designer label or art deco lettering, expect to find them priced at $15-25. *Author's collection.*

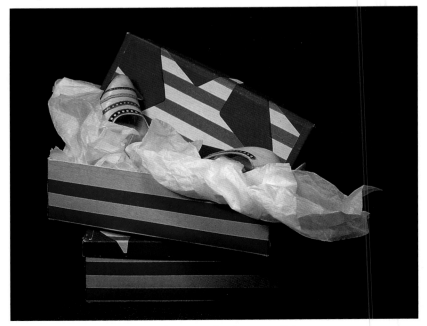

The bold graphics of the *Miss America* shoebox set off the crayon-color banding on this white kid pump. Both box and shoes date to the mid-1950s. *Courtesy of It's About Time.* Value for both: $15-25.

Paraphenalia

Shoe accouterments can be quite pretty, and add interest to any shoe collection. Choose from wooden lasts and shoetrees, ivory shoehorns, and sterling silver buttonhooks. Although vintage shoe boxes do not have quite the *cachet* as hatboxes, they can still be useful for storage and display in your closet or dressing area.

Buckles and button covers are also fun to collect. They are available in a wide range of prices, reflecting the materials and workmanship that went into their manufacture. But all of these little jewel-like accessories reflect the artistry and aesthetics of an era.

Stockings and hose are another way to expand your collecting repertoire. As worn by women, stockings influenced fashion as much as any single accessory, and more than most. Without sheer silk hosiery, hem lines would never have risen to the knee in the Roaring '20s. And *sans* fishnet hose, the mini-skirt might never have emerged, despite relaxed social mores in the Swinging '60s.

Silk stockings were originally worn by men with the short, puffed pantaloons that were correct for court attire in sixteenth century France. The mercers' guilds of Orleans recorded strict rules: the silk must be pliable enough to be twisted; tops and heels must be neatly finished; seams must be well-sewn. If black, the dye process must wait for the finished product. It was also required that each stocking weigh at least three ounces, or be confiscated!

Some readers will remember the panic women felt upon realizing that silk stockings and nylons would no longer be readily available due to the shortages of World War II. *Vogue* captured the moment in this excerpt from a tongue-in-cheek article that ran in September 1941:

> "On the heels of the U.S. embargo on Japanese silk, riots broke forth at usually serene stocking counters. Sales went up 1,000 percent. With less dignity than the Marx Brothers, women kicked, clawed, and glared their way to the disheveled salesgirls. Places which allowed a limited number of pairs to a customer found women using every device but false mustaches to get more. It might have been funny if it hadn't had a dead-earnest, nightmare quality.
>
> "This panic about a stocking-market crash was entirely unnecessary. In the first place, there are, in reserve, enough silk stockings to take care of normal demands for two months. In the second place, from present indications there will continue to be enough nylon to supply 20-25 percent of normal stocking demands. In the third place, there are beautiful cotton stockings, knitted of mercerized lisle on readjusted American machines. Finally, experts are busily working on substitutes and expect to have them ready soon."

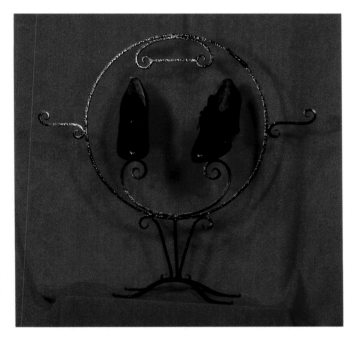

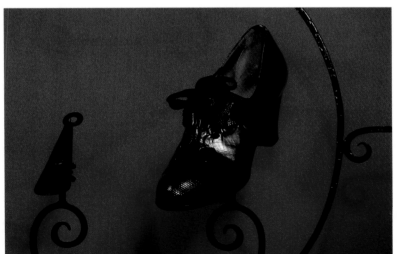

A novelty display stand circa 1910. The shoes perched like little birds, in an iron filigree cage. These black oxfords are labeled "Dickerson Arch-Relief" and they are new\old stock from approximately the same era. *Courtesy of Lindy's Shoppe.* Value: stand, $95-115; shoes, $75-95.

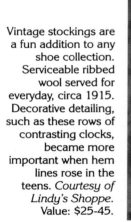

Vintage stockings are a fun addition to any shoe collection. Serviceable ribbed wool served for everyday, circa 1915. Decorative detailing, such as these rows of contrasting clocks, became more important when hem lines rose in the teens. *Courtesy of Lindy's Shoppe.* Value: $25-45.

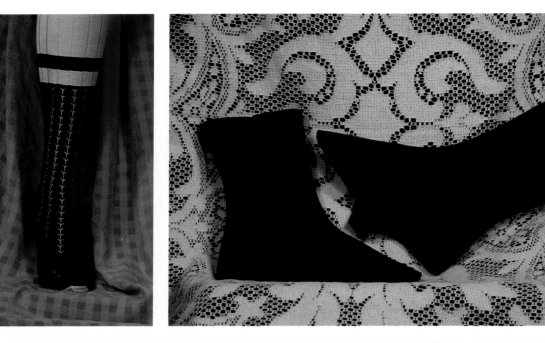

A serviceable pair of brushed-wool spats, soft as a wren's wing, circa 1895. *Courtesy of The Blue Parrot.* Value: $35-55.

206

Wooden shoetrees were often marked with the manufacturer's logo and may have been sent home with the customer as a form of advertising. *Collection of Carol Sidlow.* Value: Special.

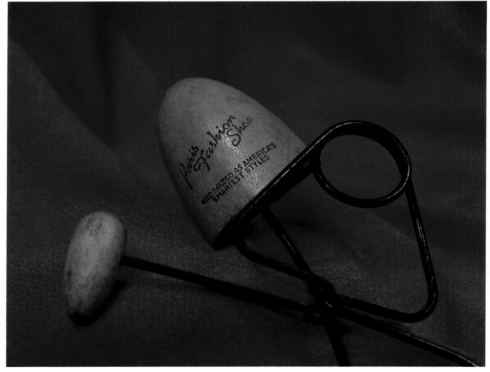

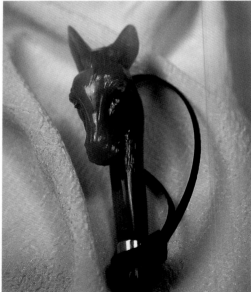

Vintage boot-and shoehorns were often works of art and would make an interesting collection in their own right. This is a mass-produced, 18-inch horn for the horsey set, circa 1950. The sculpture is molded plastic (look for examples in bone or ebony). *Courtesy of It's About Time.* Value: $15-25.

Perhaps the women were right in panicking, after all. As history tells us, the experts never did develop an acceptable substitute. True, stockings were manufactured in this country for several more years, and G. I. Joes gained quite a reputation overseas as purveyors of chocolate bars and nylons. However, by the mid-1940s women on both sides of the Atlantic were resorting to leg make-up in the summer and anklet socks in the winter. Finally, fashion magazines offered special patterns for crocheting hose at home, using yarn that could be unraveled from the best parts of old blankets and sweaters.

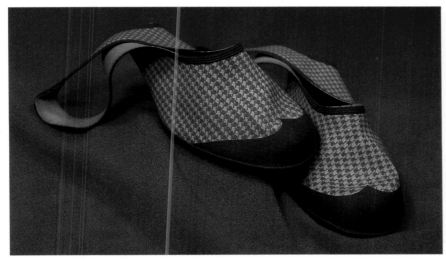

A pretty pair of red-and-white hound's-tooth rubbers, to protect slingback pumps from spring showers, circa 1949. The author was fortunate to purchase these for only $15.

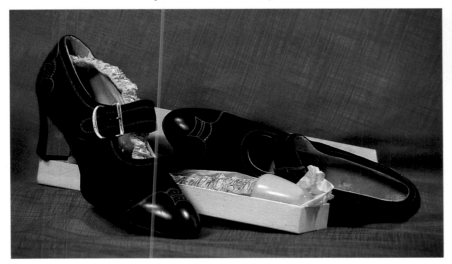

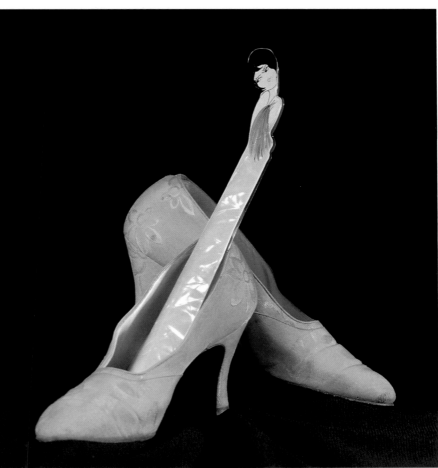

Above: Buttercup brocade opera pumps by Premier, in the pure and classic form of the late 1920s. The shoehorn is an art deco delight, from the same era. *Courtesy of Lindy's Shoppe.* Value: shoes, $75-95; horn, $45-65.

Left: Vintage yellow shoetrees keep these new\old stock shoes in shape, and they're cheerful too. The shoes are single-bar black suede with kid toecaps, in their original box, circa 1935. *Courtesy of Past Perfect.* Value: trees, $10-15; shoes, $55-75.

Showing Off

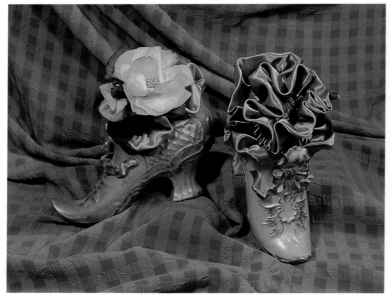

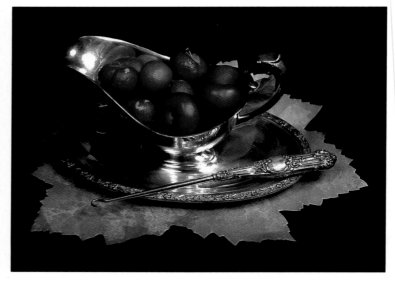

When a silver buttonhook is this pretty, let it shine in the dining room with the rest of the sterling. It's looking good enough to eat (or eat with) at the side of a silver gravy boat. *Collection of Carol Sidlow.* Value: Special.

Viola De Cou collects shoes for their intrinsic beauty and to garner new ideas for Panache, her line of custom-made boutique and boudoir accessories. "Sometimes I get so excited about a new idea that I can't sleep at night." These bisque and satin slippers were just such a project, inspired by court shoes from the late Baroque period.

Short on display space for your collectibles? Why not pair a wee pair of china slippers such as these with a cup and saucer for a tea party with elfin charm? Shoes, boots, and slippers are a popular motif in china and glass, and usually sell for under $25. *Courtesy of Rich Man, Poor Man.*

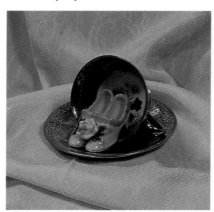

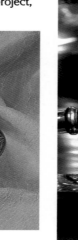

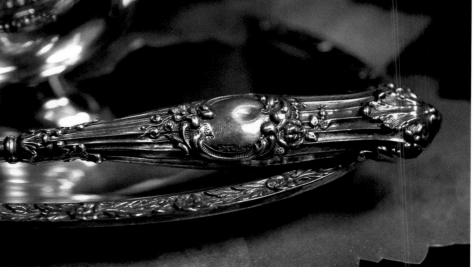

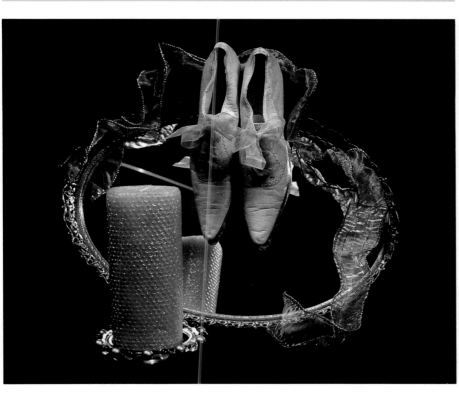

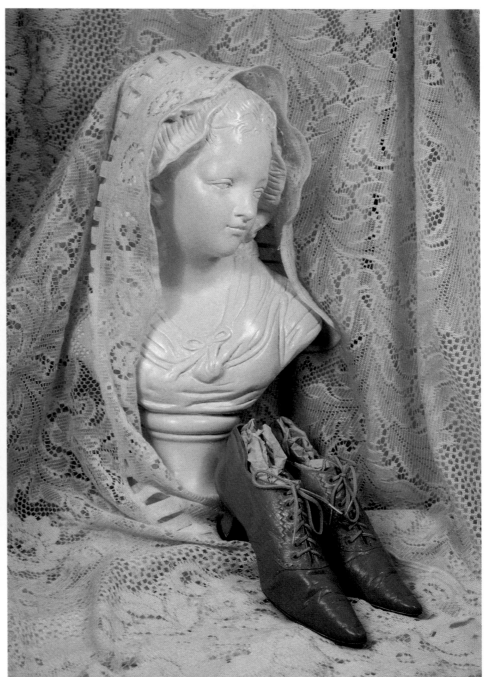

Above: Create the trendy look of a bohemian boudoir with vintage shoes, ribbons, and a filigree-framed mirror. These shoes can be dated to the mid-1800s by the "straight" soles and Louis heel. Originally white, a former owner saw fit to paint them with pink Shu Makeup! They have lost any real value, but are much enjoyed by the author nonetheless.

Right: The same pink Shu Makeup shoes are shown here, restored somewhat by a new dye job in decorous dove gray.

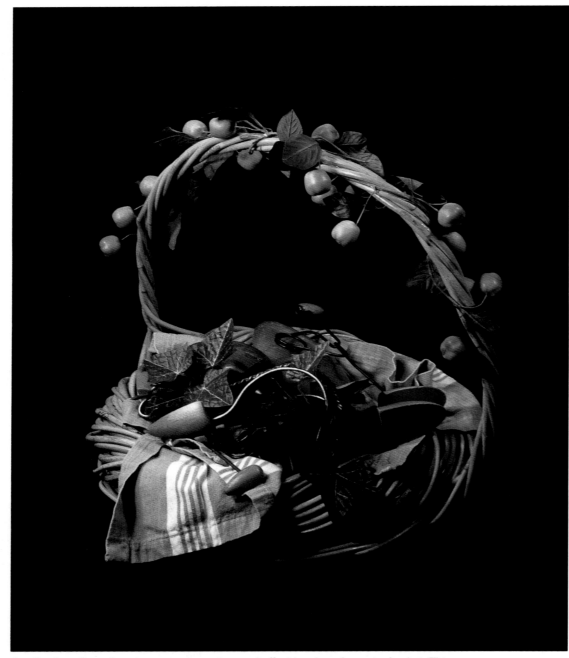

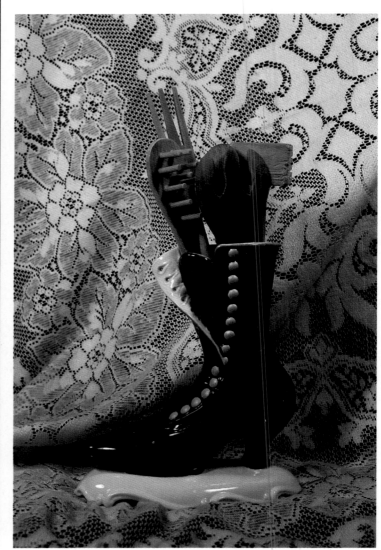

A collection of wooden shoetrees shows to good effect in a broad country basket. This could also form the base of a fruit or floral arrangement, for a summertime buffet or casual coffee table. *Collection courtesy of Romantic Notions.* Fancy shoetrees from the early 1900s sell for $35-55, their modern counterparts should be about $15.

An amusing china vase shaped like a high-button shoe would be quite at home on the sill of an old-fashioned kitchen window, holding flowers or wooden spoons, as suits your fancy. *Author's collection.* Value: $25.

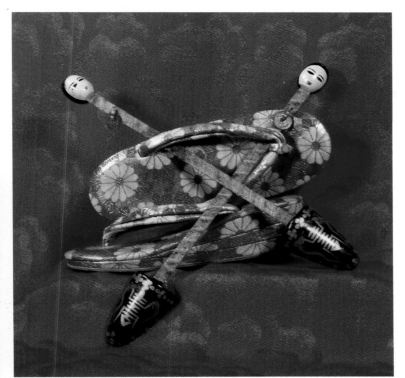

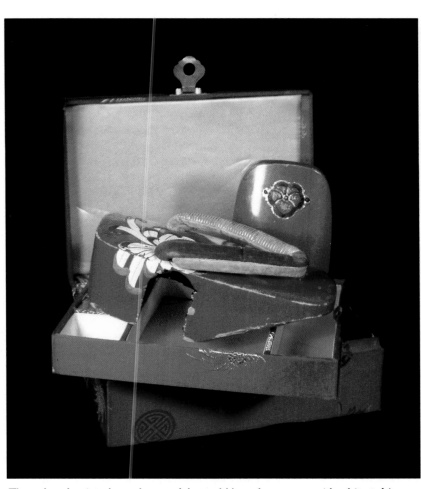

These hand-painted wooden sandals would have been worn with white *tabis* by a Japanese girl in pre-World War II Japan. The metal stud is shaped like a chrysanthemum, for good luck. *Collection of Gail Pocock.* Value: Special.

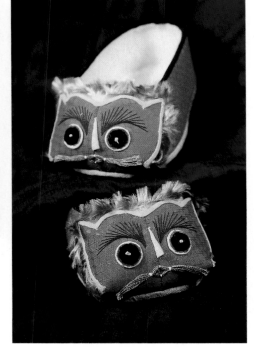

Above: Vintage shoetrees with dangling good-luck coins a winsome picture when posed with a pair of floral silk *getas. Author's collection.* Value: Special.

Left: Frisky lion-head slippers play like kittens! They were sewn by loving hands, right down to an embroidery-knot design on the soles. Since the inner cotton lining is slightly soiled, they appear to have been worn by chubby feet before they were carefully tucked away. Children's shoes can be tied together with cording and hung from a doorknob or hook (add a tartan-plaid bow for holiday charm). *Author's collection.* Value: Special.

211

Chapter X

VALUATION GUIDE

The French are undisputed leaders in the realm of *haute couture*, fashion, and style. But what of vintage clothing and its valuation? It may still be said that the French have a word for it: *laissez faire*. It was a central economic doctrine of the last century, during those days before personal income taxes and consumer price indexing. Its followers opposed government regulation of the marketplace on the assumption that consumers would properly price goods and services based on supply and demand. Roughly translated, the term itself means "what the traffic will bear." When it comes to shopping for vintage clothing, perhaps a better motto would be "buyer beware."

We have tried to give prevailing market prices for vintage shoes, based on the prices in Northern California at the time of publication. Prices in Southern California are somewhat skewed by the motion picture trade with much higher prices at certain shops that cater to the industry. Indeed, throughout California, vintage clothing shops have rented to costumers and designers for reproduction in period motion pictures. Fortunately, in most cases these acquisitions are preserved in costumer archives after filming.

Now the trend is for the vintage clothing and accessories to be purchased outright and worn by the actors and actresses.

Since prices can vary so broadly from region to region, we give a value range for the shoes shown in this book. Assume they are in good condition unless otherwise indicated (new\old stock will command a higher price). If only one shoe is shown, assume there is a pair, unless stated to be a single. Finally, assume these are the prices you will find in vintage clothing stores. If anything, these prices may be a bit low, especially as compared to special shows, but not low enough for true bargain hunters. If that means you, we recommend scouring flea markets and garage sales where prices should be even lower.

You will see the term "special" used often to denote a private collection where the owner wanted privacy on the subject of price.

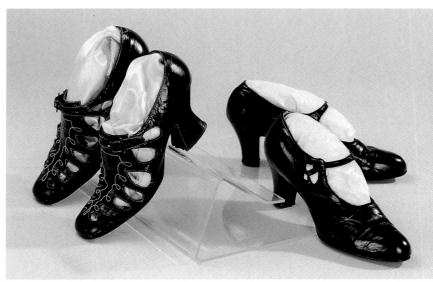

Basic black leather shoes, in a sturdy style, possibly the most popular in every era. This type of shoe can be a real bargain. *Courtesy of It's About Time.* Value: $25-35.

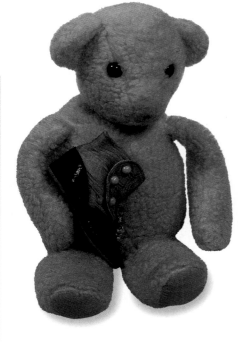

You can add "sentimental value" to any pair of children's shoes, whether worn or not. In fact, sometimes the wear just adds to the charm. Even "singles" will sell for high prices, since they still make a charming addition to a collection and display well (as shown). The bright shoe button eyes of this well-loved Teddy watch over baby's first high-button bootie from the turn-of-the-century. *Courtesy of Rich Man, Poor Man.* Value, single: $35-55.

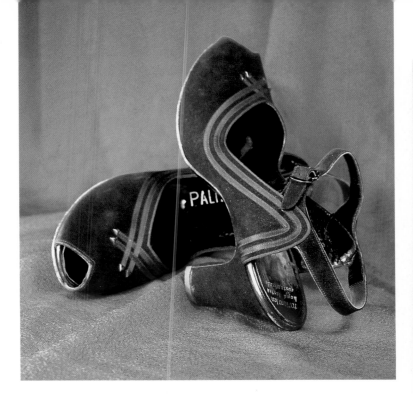

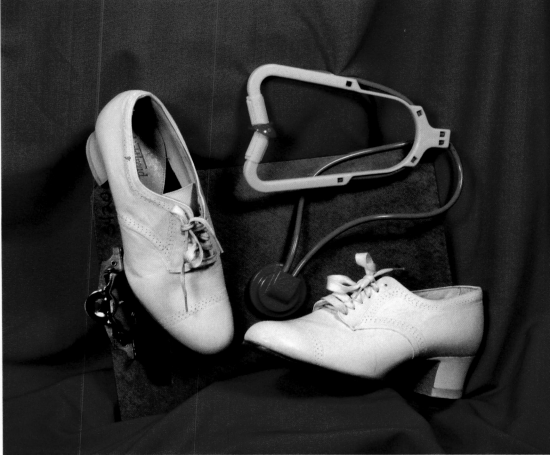

Don't step on my blue suede shoes! A brace of satin bands makes these shoes special, from Palizzio circa 1942. *Courtesy of Rhonda Barrett*. With this custom touch, the value is $35-55; otherwise, only $25-35.

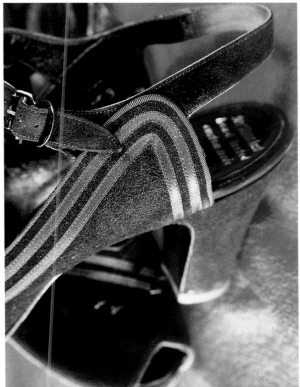

Unusual shoes are hard to value, like these nurse's oxfords in old\new stock. They may be shunned by the average shoe collector, but sought after by one who also works in the medical field. *Courtesy of Lottie Ballou*. Value: Special.

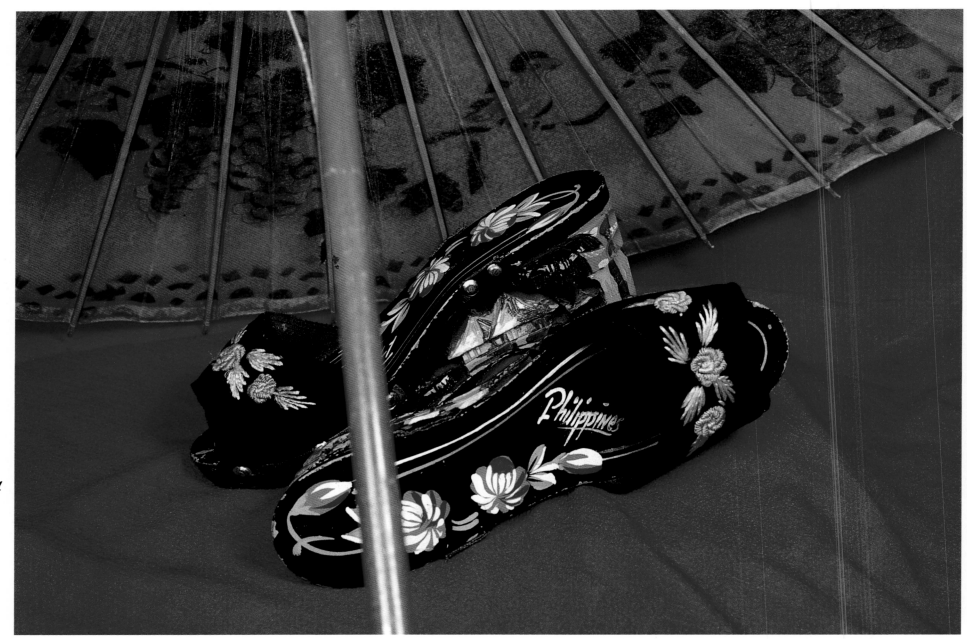

214

The elaborate hand-carved scene on these wooden platform sandals
is dazzling in polychrome paint. Typically, they are pre-World War II,
from the Philippines. *Author's collection.* Value: Special.

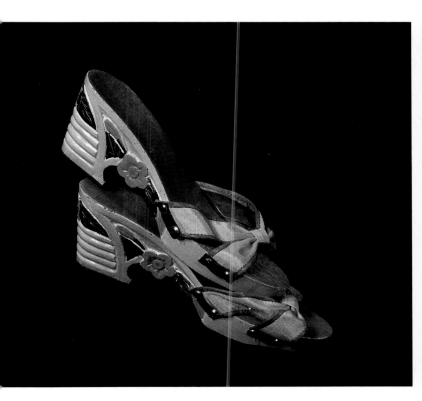

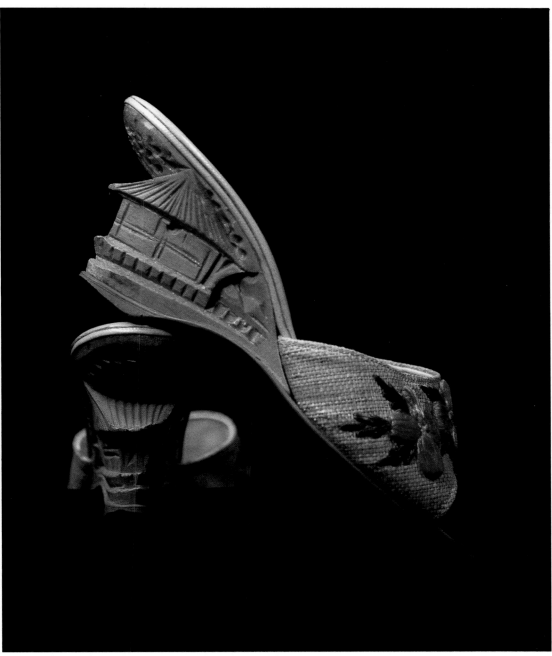

Above: Another scenic wooden sandal, with floral motif. This type of shoe makes an amusing collection, but don't expect to wear them—they are usually size 6 and under! *Author's collection.* Value: Special.

Right: The carved wedgie with raffia vamp is from the mid-1950s. Made in Hawaii, mules like this were sold to tourists to go with their newly acquired muu muus. *Courtesy of The Blue Parrot.* Value: $25-55.

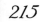

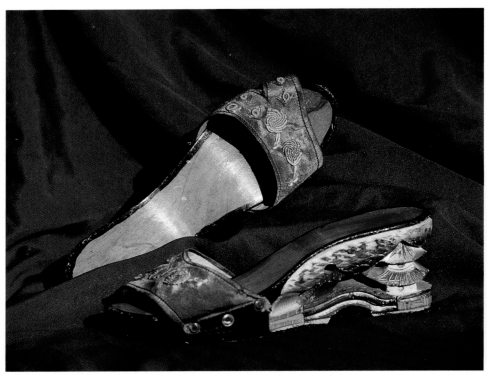

The author purchased these carved wooden platforms for $25 at a vintage clothing store in Sacramento. Later, she spied an almost identical pair priced $225, at a famous vintage emporium in the trendy Melrose district of Los Angeles. As the saying goes, you'd better shop around!

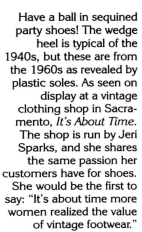

Have a ball in sequined party shoes! The wedge heel is typical of the 1940s, but these are from the 1960s as revealed by plastic soles. As seen on display at a vintage clothing shop in Sacramento, *It's About Time*. The shop is run by Jeri Sparks, and she shares the same passion her customers have for shoes. She would be the first to say: "It's about time more women realized the value of vintage footwear."

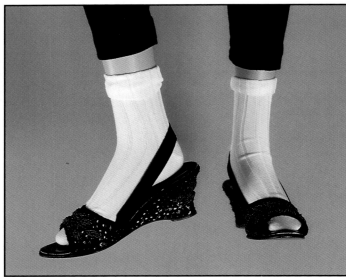

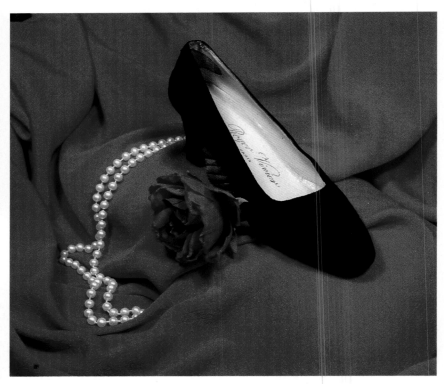

Above & opposite: You'll have to compete with museum curators to find a pair of the fanciful shoes that Roger Vivier designed for Christian Dior in the 1950s. Settle for this pair—less artistic but more wearable in cropped silk velvet—imported from Paris circa 1965. *Courtesy of Luxe.* Value: $75-95.

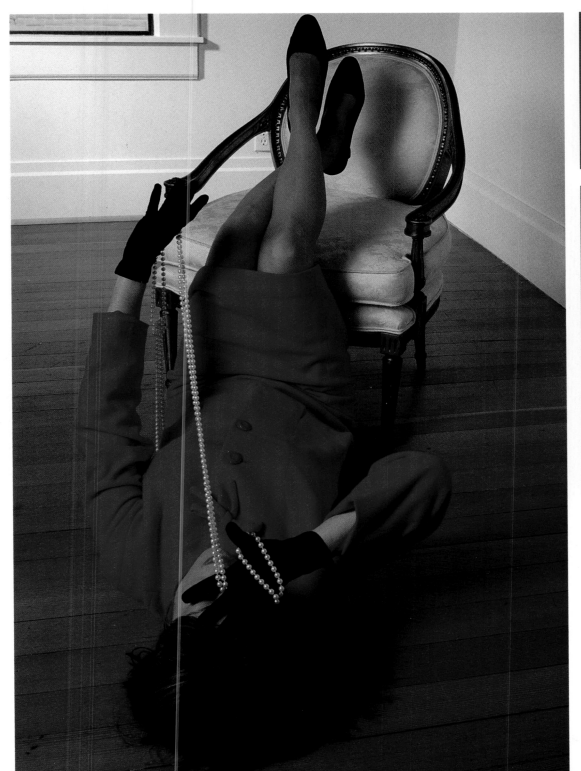

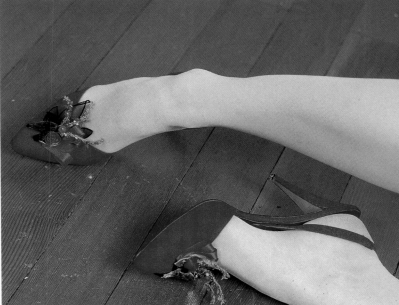

It's hard to value designer shoes that are only *slightly* vintage. Of course they are top quality, and the artistry may be so original as to render them timeless. These red slingbacks by Andrea Pfister are a good example of witty shoes from the 1980s that would still be sought after by some vintage collectors. *Collection of Laurie Gordon.* Value: Special.

Chapter XI

FOOT NOTES

The shoe as *objet d'arche*. This motif has appeared in china, glass, and metal; in velvet, cotton, and satin. It has been formed into pincushions, vases, candy dishes, hatpin holders, and pomanders. It has been printed on stationery, calendars, and post-cards. It has been stitched into pillows and enameled into brooches. The lady's slipper whispers of charm and grace; the manly boot shouts its strength. And the baby's booty is the favorite keepsake of all, murmuring a sweet lullaby to all who pause to listen.

The shoe is a symbol of rank. When the tomb of boy-king Tutankhamen was opened in 1922, among his personal effects was a pair of peaked sandals fashioned from embossed gold. When he was buried, in the year 1343 BC, the Egyptians had a special hieroglyph for sandal, which looked like an oval with a inverted "V" on the inside.

The shoe is a homily. How many expressions of sympathy, envy, anger, awe, and love can we trace to the powerful footprint of shoes on our culture? Foot in mouth and two left feet; well-heeled, down-at-the-heels, and cool your heels. You can put down your foot; get on equal footing, and bet your boots. But can you fill his boots, and think on your feet? Are you head over heels in love with shoes?

The vintage shoe is an object of passion. As art historian George Kubler observed, "objects are portions of arrested happening." We say that the occupations and aspirations of another time are frozen in the form of a shoe, as an *objet d'arche*.

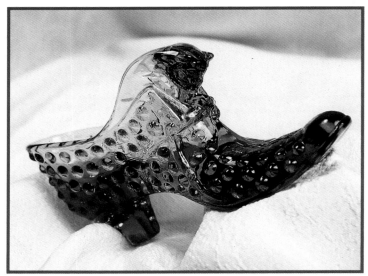

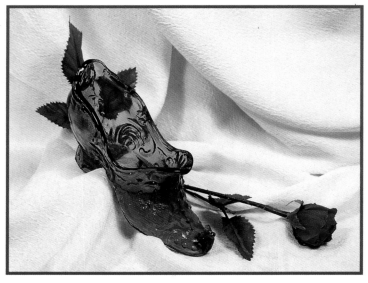

Sandwich glass slippers were a highly popular bibelot in the mid-century. They were made in a full range of clear colors, plus milk glass and hobnail glass. You can easily find them in antique malls and flea markets for $15-35. *Author's collection.*

GLOSSARY

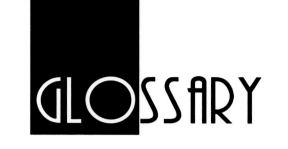

Adelaide: Ladies' fashion boots, side-laced, from the early to mid-1800s.

Argenté: A silvered over glaze, usually on kidskin.

Ballet slipper: A flat shoe with shallow vamp and grosgrain cording at the throat to look like it would cinch at the vamp like the suede-soled practice slippers worn by ballerinas.

Bar: A strap across the instep which helps hold the shoe on the foot. The bar may be single or double. If single, this style is more popularly known as the Mary Jane.

Barrette: A style of shoe closed by multiple straps across the instep buttoned at the side or in the middle. Likewise, a style of boot closed by the same type of multiple straps across the instep and continuing up the shin. Usually referring to an evening style with beadwork on the barrettes and mother-of-pearl buttons for closure.

Boot: The basic shoe form in leather or rubber extended up the leg for protection and warmth. Boots usually end at ankle, mid-calf, or knee.

Bottine: Women's elastic-sided boot, first designed for Queen Victoria, generally in a natural fawn leather with black toe-cap.

Bridge shoe: A dressy slipper for hostess and at-home wear, named for the habit of bridge players to slip on comfortable shoes while at the card table.

Brocade: A rich silk of any color, thickly textured with raised patterns in gold or silver.

Brocatelle: A stiff brocade with raised patterns in high relief.

Brogue: Stout leather walking shoe of Irish origin, originally soled with hobnails.

Bulldogs: Style of shoe or boot with high, blunt toe boxing. Popular for men and children at the turn-of-the-century.

Buskin: A calf-length boot that laced up the front with a height-enhancing heel, originally worn by Greek actors. See *cuissarde*.

Chopines: Shoes elevated shoes on extremely thick cork soles, often 6-8 inches high, associated with the courtesans of eighteenth century Venice.

Clock: An ornamental figure on the ankle or side of a stocking or sock.

Clogs: A shoe, sandal, or overshoe having a thick wooden sole. See *sabots*.

Cording: Fabric or leather sewn over a string, used to trim the throat of a shoe.

Court shoe: A plain, closed shoe with medium to high heels. See opera pump.

Counter: The very back piece of a shoe, where the heel of the foot ends.

Cuissarde: A leather or suede over-the-knee boot, usually laced up the side.

Décolleté: Having a low-cut throat line, so as to expose the cleavage.

d'Orsay: A graceful pump with almond toe, scooped vamp, and low-waisted heel, named for its designer Count d'Orsay.

Duckbills: Cloth or leather shoes with a single-bar closure and flat soles, so named because of their extremely wide toe-boxing.

Espadrille: A flat shoe with a cloth upper and rope sole.

Felt: A dense flat-knapped fabric, formed by soaking and pressing the fibers of wool or fur, until they interlock.

Gaiters: An ankle covering of canvas, linen, or leather worn principally by men. They buttoned down the side and were often strapped to the undersole of the shoe.

Garters: A ribbon, elasticized cuff, clip, or other device used to hold up stockings.

Glacé: Any over glaze, adding a subtle gloss to dyed or natural kidskin and other leathers. See argenté and pearlized.

Guilloche: A decorative treatment on metal, formed from interlaced bands with the openings filled by enamel. Referred to as "machine-turned" when the bands are geometric.

Grosgrain: A type of textured ribbon formed by close-set, horizontal ribbing. Known as Petersham ribbon in England.

Gusset: The triangular piece of elastic set into the side of boots in the nineteenth century .

Getas: Stilted wooden platforms that strap to the foot and raise it above dirt and mud, as worn in ancient Japan.

Faille: A middleweight, ribbed fabric with a slight luster. It is usually woven from silk, cotton, or rayon.

Heel breast: The flat portion of a heel that faces the sole and may be lined with the same leather as the sole.

Heel waist: The middle portion of a heel, referring to a slight dip or curve.

Huaraches: A flat-heeled sandal with the upper formed by interlaced leather straps, indigenous to Mexico.

Insole lining: The paper or cloth lining that covers the inside part of a shoe, and on which the label is often stamped or sewn.

Instep: That part of the foot that runs from ankle to toes, above the arch.

Jacquard: A type of woven fabric with intricate figural or geometric raised patterns in the same color, or in the reverse color when a weave is two-faced.

Juliet Shoe: A slipper worn by ladies of the leisure class in the early 1900s. It was worn "at home" and is a forerunner of the "bridge shoe." It had a low, waisted heel and cut-away sides. The vamp and quarters were elongated to extend up the ankle.

Laces: Cords or strings used to draw together two edges of a garment or shoe, typically passed through metal-framed holes or "grommets."

Last: A shape of wood or metal that conforms to the measurement of a person's foot, or a standardized foot size. The last must be shaped to accommodate a certain height of heel, and a separate last is required for the heel.

Lastex: A stretchy, synthetic material that could be woven into fabric and leather for elasticity.

Lamé: A gold or silver fabric woven with metallic threads.

Louis heel: A waisted heel, either high or low, named after King Louis XIV of France.

Mule: A backless slipper, originally flat-soled, worn in the boudoir circa 1500–1700. It developed a heel circa 1800–1900, and was then worn as a casual shoe. An enduring style, it is currently worn with any heel height, for any occasion.

One-off: Slang for the practice of making shoes for just one customer, with a custom last.

Opera pump: A plain, graceful pump with medium or high heel. See Court shoe.

Oxfords: Originally a man's shoe of the late nineteenth century, with ties that laced at the instep and around the ankles. Adopted by women in the early twentieth century, now it stands for any laced-up walking shoe.

Pattens: High wooden platforms that strapped to the shoe, mostly worn by ladies in the 1600–1800s to keep their feet and skirts clear of the dirty streets.

Pearlized: An ivory over glaze to dyed or natural kidskin and other leathers.

Piping: Thicker than cording, but similar, a type of trim used to cover a seam or set off the contrast between different pieces of the shoe.

Poulaine: Flat shoe with an extremely long, pointed toe worn by men in the Middle Ages. The style was condemned by the church for its phallic appearance.

Princess: A style of slim and tapered heel, about 2 inches in height, typically used for the simple pump or "court shoe."

Pump: The basic shoe shape. Closed at toe and heel, with a medium to high heel. Proper for day and evening, depending on the material and trim.

Pyrograph: A heat treatment for dyed or natural leather, creating an embossed design.

Quarters: That part of the shoe that covers the sides of the foot, running from heel (counter) to vamp.

Rosette: A circle of shirred ribbon, or a ribbon bow, often used to decorate shoes for both sexes in the seventeenth century.

Saddle shoe: A flat-soled spectator with contrasting sides or "saddles." Popular since the '20s, but most often associated with American teenagers of the '50s. Traditionally in white buckskin with tan saddles and red rubber soles.

Sabots: The wooden shoes often associated with little Dutch girls. Hand-carved from blocks of balsa wood and worn by peasants in Medieval Europe. They were revived during the shortages of World War II and are still worn today by working-class men and women, especially in the Netherlands.

Sandal: Known now as any open-toe shoe in leather or other materials, sandals may also feature open sides and heel and be held on by straps at the toe (thongs) or across the instep. Adapted from the ancient Roman *solea*, or a leather sole strapped to the foot.

Satin: A type of fabric, usually woven from silk or rayon, with a glossy surface and a matt backside.

Shank: The arch support, built into a well-made shoe as part of the inner construction. Vintage shoes often used steel arch supports; now they are often foam rubber.

Shagreen: A luxury material, green-gray in color with a lustrous sheen, that is processed by hand from sharkskin. Popular in the 1920s and 1930s for shoes, belts, wallets, boxes, and any other item that could be formed from leather.

Shantung: A textured Chinese silk woven from coarse yarn.

Shoe: An outer covering for the foot, usually made of leather, with a thick or stiff sole and an attached heel.

Shoehorn: A scoop-like device to help the heel slip into a tight shoe or boot; originally, whittled from a cow-horn.

Shoetree: A foot-shaped wooden form, or oval wooden shapes held by a flexible strip of metal, that may be inserted into a shoe or boot to preserve its shape.

Silk: A fine yet durable fabric woven from the lining of a silkworm cocoon. It originated in ancient China and was a key commodity for export to Europe in early East-West trading.

Slingback: A closed-toe shoe without rear quarters, held on at the back with a strap.

Slipper: A light, low-cut shoe that is easily slipped on over the foot and is used for undress. Also, any delicate lady's shoe.

Sneakers: A flat canvas sport shoe with rubber sole, laced up over the tongue. It is derived from the English gym-shoe of the teens and '20s. The modern sneaker, based on a prototype developed by Nike in the '60s, is worn in all seasons and for all reasons.

Sole: The bottom of any footwear. Usually of leather or rubber, this is the part that touches the ground.

Spanish heel: A graceful waisted heel, usually 2 to 3 inches high.

Spats: A short gaiter covering the lower ankle and upper foot, usually of linen or felt. Both stylish and practical, spats were popular with men and women at the turn-of-the-century.

Spectator: Any two-tone shoe for men or women. Traditionally of white or cream leather with black or brown at heel and toe, it was designed to keep wet grass from staining the shoes worn with summer whites by spectators at a polo, cricket, or tennis match. In Britain this style is dubbed "co-respondent."

Stacked heel: Referring to the process of manufacture, from thin slices of wood that are stacked like pancakes then glued together and shaped. May be any height.

Tabis: Soft white cotton socks with a separation for the big toe, like mittens for the foot, worn for warmth in lieu of shoes in ancient Japan; still worn indoors in modern Japan.

Tassel: A pendent ornament made from bunched strips of leather or twisted yarn, fastened at one end. Often used as a zipper-pull on shoes and boots.

Thai silk: Slubbed silk, like Shantung, but dyed and woven to create an iridescent sheen.

Thong: Minimal sandals in leather or rubber, held on the foot by a "thong" strap gripped between the toes.

Throat: The top line of a shoe, usually trimmed with piping.

Toe box: The structured part of the lower vamp that covers the toes, especially referring to shape (square, pointed, almond).

Uppers: The upper part of a shoe consisting of counter, quarter, vamp, and toe boxing.

Vamp: The upper part of a boot or shoe, extending from the ankle to the toe, in front.

Wedgies: Shoes with a wedge-shaped heel that extends the length of the sole. The arch may be filled in or pierced. Originally shaped from cork or balsa wood. Typically, the wedge sole is covered with the same leather or fabric as the shoe.

Welt: The seam that connects the upper to the sole, or any extra piece of fabric or leather that reinforces seams.

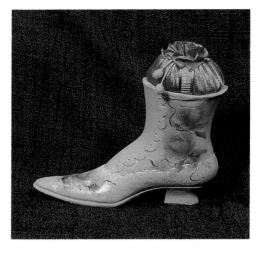

SELECTED BIBLIOGRAPHY

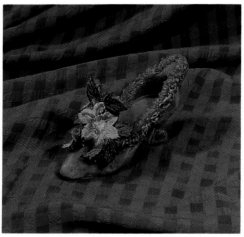

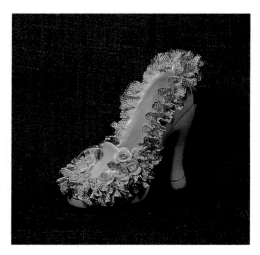

Boccardi, Luciana. *Party Shoes*. Modena, Italy: Zanfi Editori with Bella Casa, 1993.

Girotti, Eugenia. *Footwear (La Calzatura)*. San Francisco: Chronicle Books, 1997.

Lawlor, Laurie. *Where Will This Shoe Take You?*. New York City: Walker & Co., 1996.

Lobenthal, Joel. *Radical Rags: Fashions of the Sixties*. New York City: Abbeville Press, 1990.

Martin, Richard. *The St. James Fashion Encyclopedia: A Survey of Style from 1945 to the Present*. Detroit, Michigan: Visible Ink Press, 1997.

McDowell, Colin. *Shoes: Fashion and Fantasy*. London: Thames & Hudson Ltd., 1989.

Mulvagh, June. *Vogue History of 20th Century Fashion*. New York City: Viking; London: Penguin Inc., 1988.

O'Keefe, Linda. *Shoes*. New York City: Workman Publishing Co. Inc., 1996.

Probert, Cristina. *Shoes in Vogue Since 1910*. New York City: Abbeville Press with Conde Nast, 1981.

Sunshine, Linda & Tiegreen. *Mary: A Passion for Shoes*. Kansas City, Kansas: Andrews & McMeel with Universal Press Syndicate Co., 1995.

Trasko, Mary. *Heavenly Soles: Extraordinary 20th Century Shoes*. New York City: Abbeville Press, 1989.

INDEX

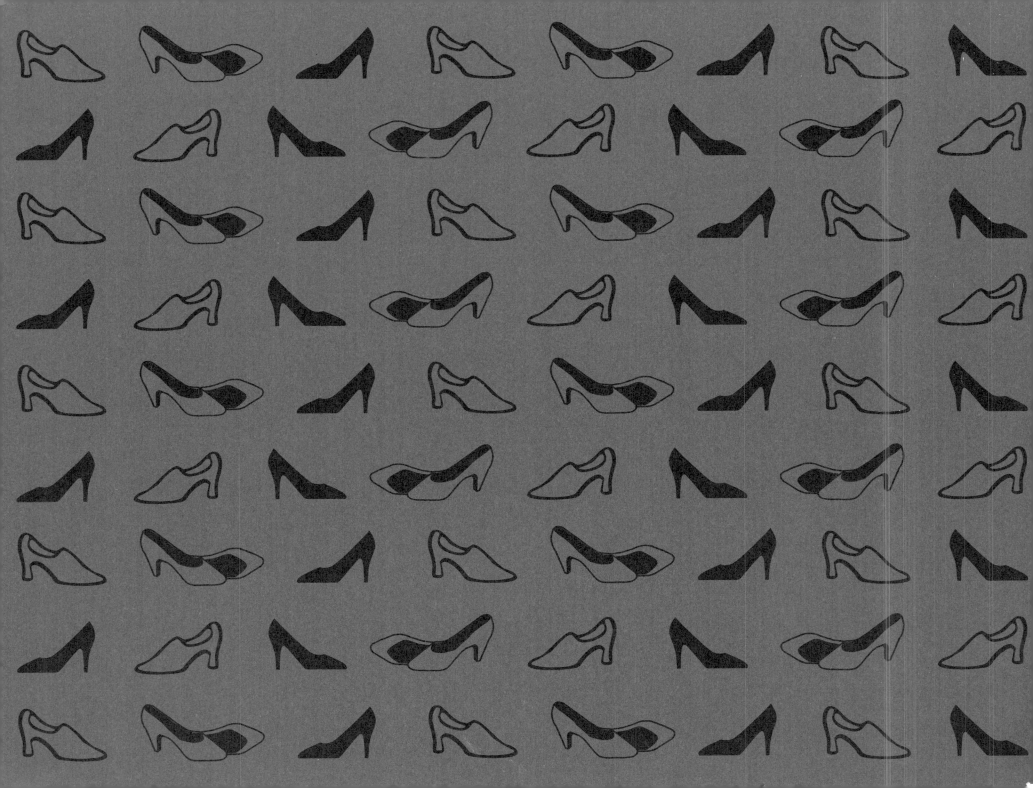